MW00795168

COCHLEAR
IMPLANT BASICS

*What a Candidate for a Cochlear Implant Needs to Know
Including Twenty-five Interviews with Candidates, Recipients,
Surgeons and Other Professionals*

RICHARD POCKER

Copyright © 2021
RICHARD POCKER
COCHLEAR IMPLANT BASICS
What a Candidate for a Cochlear Implant Needs to Know
Including Twenty-five Interviews with Candidates, Recipients,
Surgeons and Other Professionals

All rights reserved.

No part of this publication may be reproduced, distributed, or transmitted in any form or by any means, including photocopying, recording, or other electronic or mechanical methods, without the prior written permission of the publisher, except in the case of brief quotations embodied in critical reviews and certain other non-commercial uses permitted by copyright law.

RICHARD POCKER

Printed in the United States of America
First Printing 2021
First Edition 2021

ISBN: 979-8-9853613-0-8

10 9 8 7 6 5 4 3 2 1

Creator and Producer of Cochlearimplantbasics.com
Website Designed and Maintained by Infanisrael@gmail.com
Instagram: infanisrael

This book is dedicated to my wife, Beth, who stood by me through decades of my Years of Silence. Only with her love and support was I able to obtain the gift of hearing with cochlear implants and fulfill my mission of helping others find a way out of the isolation of deafness.

TABLE OF CONTENTS

Preface to Cochlear Implant Basics

Chris woke up one morning deaf in her right ear. She was thirty-two years old. She had a very good job where hearing was essential for socializing with donors. She was in a panic but held on to her position until it was no longer possible.

David was a sportswriter for a newspaper. His hearing loss caused him to make embarrassing mistakes when he collected scores or names on the phone.

Sarah and Michelle are parents who discovered their children suffered from severe hearing loss and their developmental skills were at a severe risk.

Nanette was a lead singer for a world-renown group who suffered from a genetic hearing loss and had to withdraw from her career.

Mary Beth, a teacher of the deaf, found herself with a severe hearing loss too but took lessons from the children in her classes.

All these stories, and more are captured in these interviews.

While all hearing losses are as unique as our fingerprints, what they have in common is every one of these people eventually turned to the scientific wonder of a cochlear implant to find a way out of the isolation and the crisis that deafness brings.

This post received from a cochlear implant recipient in the UK, in response to the podcast in chapter 25 about grieving for hearing loss, sums up best the entire concept behind the need for support that Cochlear Implant Basics supplies. As W.B. put it:

Hi Richard, A great, encouraging, and supportive read.

I was suddenly deafened and freely admit I grieved! Folks would say, but you've just lost your hearing! I said if you suddenly lost your right arm, would you miss it?, wouldn't you be angry you are not able to do things with one arm, you could easily manage with both arms? Wouldn't you be sad at the future adjustment to be a one arm person? Who is queuing up to lose a sense or a body part because it's a fantastic idea?

I'm one of the ones who toughed it out, as no counselling available in my area in the UK. Using a certain amount of, anger, stubbornness, frustration, humor and if the situation called for it 'faking it' and bare faced lying! It was a case of here's your cochlear implant, do the exercises.

Audiologist had no idea when it will get better enough to help to retain my job, whilst I'm pooping bricks terrified I may lose it.

Your life hasn't flashed by before your eyes....it just stopped.

Audiologist had no idea, if or when I would be able to hear a conversation without asking for multiple repeats. Here's the address of the big D Community Centre, join it, may help. We will arrange your flashing doorbell and sonic shake bed smoke alarm. Happy hearing, off you trot.

I'm very lucky my friends/family/colleagues continue to adjust and be supportive of my hearing loss.

I'm a hearing person who accepts, I am a deaf person who hears via a cochlear implant. Took me a while, but I finally got there!

Cochlear Implant Basics is a website for candidates, recipients, and their families and friends.

If you or a loved one is profoundly hard of hearing, newly deaf, or have experienced sudden hearing loss. Here are the stories that tell how receiving a cochlear implant can be a life-changing event.

This site is not medical advice, nor is it brand specific nor is the site sponsored by any company or organization.

You will meet recipients who faced hearing loss situations, and hearing aids could no longer provide comprehension of speech or music. They share the stories of how they lost their hearing, their struggles with growing isolation from their family and friends, their inability to compete in the world of business, their difficulties of navigating air travel without hearing, how the joy of music disappeared, and the panic of not being able to use a telephone to contact 9-1-1 to get aid for a loved one.

Disclaimer: THIS BOOK IS NOT OFFERING MEDICAL ADVICE. CONSULT YOUR OWN HEALTH CARE PROVIDER.

PREFACE TO EXPANDED EDITION

Since the publication of Cochlear Implant Basics in December 2021, the need for more topics became evident.

This new edition contains interviews that follow up such as the one with Lou Ferrigno, captured more than a year after his initial activation. Isabella Rodriguez, a Cochlear BAHA recipient (now upgraded to Osia) was a missing topic in the first edition. Doctor Herb Silverstein, a world authority on Meniere's and hyperacusis is included as well as Rebecca Alexander, a cochlear implant user who suffers with Ushers syndrome which has left her deaf and blind.

There were two inspirational cochlear implant recipients with stories that remind us that hearing loss is not the end of your dreams to accomplish whatever you want to. Mike Dailey, a bilateral CI recipient who is an EMT or Oliva Rose Allen, a certified pilot. They are a reminder that hearing loss is not an insurmountable barrier to greatness.

The options for rehabilitation resources has been expanded. Rehabilitation is the key to getting optimal results from a cochlear implant. The more you put into it, the better you will hear.

Don't be robbed of full participation in life. If you are on the fence about getting a cochlear implant, keep in mind that by changing nothing, nothing changes.

Carpe diem.

Sarasota

April 2023

Introduction Cochlear Implant Basics

Imagine suddenly losing your hearing and going stone deaf. Speech, music, environmental sounds; all gone.

Terrifying isn't it?

It happened to me, and I spent 35 years in total silence until I received bilateral cochlear implants just before my 65th birthday. During those decades of silence, I had no comprehension of speech, or music and not an inkling of what was going on around me.

Since being activated with bilateral cochlear implants in January 2016 I have been on a mission to help others get out of the isolation of deafness. My website cochlearimplantbasics.com has been one of the tools I use. I have moved hundreds of candidates forward.

Cochlear implants are not magic bullets. There is a need to rehabilitate to get your brain to understand sound. We hear with our brain, not our ears, is a common refrain. After healing from surgery, the cochlear implant recipient is activated by a specialized audiologist. Depending on multiple factors such as the length of deafness prior to surgery and individual differences, activation day may range from hearing beeps and whistles to comprehension of speech. There is no way to predict, and the recipient needs to attend with low expectation but knowing with dedication to performing hearing exercises, they will improve.

With rehabilitation, I have gone from zero speech recognition to 85%. Music took a bit longer to return. Today all sounds are natural to me. I enjoy socializing, listening to music and can use a phone without hesitation.

The twenty-five interviews in Cochlear Implant Basics have minor editing for clarity. They cover a wide range of experiences of different types of hearing loss, from candidates, recipients, surgeons, and other professionals who lend their expertise to the subject.

Disclaimer: THIS BOOK IS NOT OFFERING MEDICAL ADVICE. CONSULT YOUR OWN HEALTH CARE PROVIDER.

PART ONE

CANDIDATES AND RECIPIENTS

CHAPTER 1 RICHARD POCKER

ENDING 35 YEARS OF SILENCE

Richard: My name is Richard Pocker and we're in Osprey, Florida at Daddy O's Record store. One of my favorite places. And today is May 31st, 2019.

Chris: Let's talk a little bit about your hearing loss.

Richard: Sure.

Chris: Tell me, was it health issues?

Richard: I had scarlet fever when I was five, and they never knew if the loss was caused by the medication or whether it was caused by the scarlet fever itself. It's never been determined, but I had a loss for about two or three years. My parents noticed something was wrong by the time I was seven, so I went through a whole process and evaluation, and I was set up with a hearing aid. It was a big box with a wire running up to my ear, and that's how it started. I wore hearing aids for thirty years.

Chris: Had your family had any history of hearing loss?

Richard: There was absolutely none. There was no background, my sister's fine, there's no hearing loss on either side of the family. It was probably the disease or the medication. We'll never know.

Chris: When you were a kid, did you start wearing hearing aids then?

Richard: I wore the box hearing aids, and I was uncomfortable. It's a very difficult thing to be a kid with this big thing sticking out of your ear and a box. It was difficult, but what could you do?

Chris: Were they effective?

Richard: They must have been, I mean it gave me some hearing. I could function in school, and I guess I could play sports, but I just had to take them out. You couldn't play sports with hearing aids in those days. Perspiration would knock them out in a moment.

Chris: As you went into high school and college, how did you cope in those environments?

Richard: High school was difficult because my high school had a requirement for language. You had to take a foreign language, and I took French because my father insisted on French. At midterm, I had a 16 out of 100, and I already developed ulcers and the teacher scared the hell out of me, so I dropped it and I managed to get the high school to agree that mathematics is a language. That's how I got through. And when I got to college, I was already bilateral and my coping mechanism there was to be the best note taker of the textbooks. I could outline the textbooks like crazy and I always found the best note taker in every classroom, and by exchanging those notes I managed to graduate Cum laude. It was difficult, but I did it. I got through.

Chris: Then there was the transition into the workplace, can you talk a little about the jobs you held?

Richard: I'm a retired third-generation picture framer and art gallery owner, my grandfather started the business. So, I started working when I was 12. I knew the business very, very well. There's no question that the hearing handicap made it harder because customers don't want to work

COCHLEARIMPLANTBASICS.COM

with someone who's not functioning fully, and somehow, I got through that, but I had total hearing loss when I was 30. I was riding up town on the bus after seeing a client, and my hearing in my right ear went. By the time I got to the end of the ride, there was no hearing in the right ear. And about a month later, my wife and I were in the movies and my left ear went.

Richard: It was just gone, that was like total loss. I couldn't wear a hearing aid anymore; I passed the threshold, and it was it. Fini. And you go through depression, and your family goes nuts, and my son was only about four years old at the time and he was putting together all his toys trying to make an invention to help daddy get his hearing back. There's no question, the support from the family was tremendous. I probably couldn't have made it without it. So eventually, guess what? You get some therapy, and you get over it. You move on, you can't dwell in that forever.

Chris: You could not use the telephone?

Richard: I could not use the telephone, I had to have people make calls for me. And when I lost my hearing, this is back around 1980, the fax machines were new, and I had to make my suppliers buy fax machines. Back then, they were about $1000 a piece and the roll paper would curl up, so everybody was resentful. My overseas suppliers used Telex, and I'm probably the last living operator of a Western Union telex machine left. I had my own telex address just like Have Gun Will Travel, where you, wire, Paladin San Francisco, I had a telex address, which was wire Pock Frames New York, so I knew how to do that.

Richard: The computer and email were coming along, and they were a godsend, no question. But telephones were impossible. I tried TTY's, the conversations were just impossible to do, so people had to make phone calls for me. I had 25 employees, I was growing my business, eventually I had seven locations. I had manufacturing, and guess what? You have to run three times harder than anybody else just to stay in place, but I did it.

Chris: Hearing loss was probably exhausting, just getting up in the morning-

Richard: Incredibly exhausting, incredibly exhausting. I would go home and just fall asleep on the living room floor. Matter of fact, I like to tell people that I was growing the art publishing business at the time. I had to do five to seven trade shows a year, and I had to do all lip reading. And the hardest ones in the world would be Atlanta, because I had to read that southern accent all day long, and I'd go back to my room, and I would just cry and fall on the floor asleep. It was very exhausting.

Chris: Did you teach yourself to read lips, or did you ever take a course?

Richard: It was something that came to me naturally. My mom took me to a speech therapist when I was very young, and Dr. Penn would teach me lip reading and he would also teach me enunciation. I still remember, he had these little paper balls he used to blow up from the Japanese stores, and you had to blow the ball across the table. He had his techniques; it was very good. That's why I could speak, I could learn to speak. The problem about when you lose your hearing completely, you can't regulate your voice. It was a problem because I had to watch facial cues to see if I was talking too loudly, or if people were leaning towards me, I knew I was speaking too softly. It was impossible to regulate your voice that way. So, that was the problem of business when you're deaf.

Chris: As the years went on, you developed all these coping mechanisms, kind of creatively actually, but then along came the concept of a cochlear implant.

Richard: That was there, but back in the 80s it was very primitive. My love was music, and I knew back then, or at least I had the conception back then, that the cochlear implants were not made for music whatsoever and I was kind of waiting for science to catch up and find a cure for my deafness.

I waited close to 35 years. I did not have a cochlear implant till just before my 65th birthday. I must tell you, therefore I love this shop, because music's come back 100%. I wear bilateral Cochlear implants, so all the sound is coming through them, and the music is just as natural as I remember when I was young.

Chris: You go to music performances?

Richard: I go to concerts. One of the great things about the implants I'm wearing, by Cochlear, the Nucleus 7, I have so many ways to adjust the sound. Originally, I was implanted with the Nucleus 6. The Nucleus 7 came out about a year and a half after that, and I paid for the upgrade, and it was so worth it. The sound is so robust and so natural, so I can go to a concert, and I have a way to adjust the sensitivity, or the base and the treble, I can adjust the direction that my sound is coming from, and it's just incredible.

Chris: So that's an interesting point, that you can get a certain type of processor but there's no reason you can't upgrade to the next technology,

Richard: That was the whole point, the reason why I chose Cochlear, is what's on the inside stays there. You have one operation I've been told is good for 74 years, so my next operation is 2100, and the surgeon hasn't been born yet. But the internal processor always stays the same. It's the external processor, this is the Nucleus 7, as they upgrade, technology advances. It will always work with what's inside of my head. In fact, I have one friend I met who was implanted ages ago, he's now on his 5th generation of a cochlear implant. It just keeps going on, he just puts a new one on the outside.

Chris: Tell us a little bit about the day of the surgery.

Richard: The surgery was scary. I put it off for five months after I agreed to do it. Now, originally when I came to Florida, I saw the hearing aids at Costco and said maybe something's improved in 30 years, so I have an appointment with them and I go get a hearing test, the guy says to me

"You're deaf as a post, there's nothing we can do for you." And it was a couple days later I was in the gym, and I ran into somebody wearing a cochlear implant, so I asked them for some information. I went to see the clinic here, and yes of course I was qualified, but I was so scared I went for a second opinion and the second doctor said to me "Why don't you do two of them at the same time?" I go "What? Are you out of your mind?" But I went home, and I thought about it, and the next day I said "fine, let's go ahead and do two at once."

Richard: Bilateral surgery is rare, but I was lucky enough to find the surgeon that was willing to do two at the same time, and my insurance company was willing to cover it. One of the things I did was before my 65th birthday, before I went on Medicare, I still had private insurance. Medicare would cover one at a time, but my private insurance took two at the same time.

Chris: Good call. How many days or weeks was it after that until you were activated?

Richard: I waited five weeks, usually people can wait three. I decided to do five because one thing when you get a cochlear implant, I'd like to remind people, you are in charge. Don't have to take the doctor or the audiologist's word for anything. I mean they are the authority figure, but if you're not feeling up to it, just delay it. Do whatever you have to, make sure you're in charge of the whole process.

Chris: That's good advice. So how has the cochlear implant changed your life?

Richard: Without a cochlear implant ... matter of fact I was at a party the other week. We're at long tables with people and somebody asked me about them, and I said, "Well I was deaf for 35 years, I only got my hearing back three years ago." So, they say "Wow, what would you have done before the cochlear implant?" I said, "I wouldn't be sitting here." Part of a hearing loss is the isolation you go through. Now, when I lost all my hearing yes, there were some friends fell by the wayside. They did not want to put up with hearing loss, they did not want to have to put up with talking to me in a special way or whatever. And that hurt, but you find out who your friends are.

Richard: Fortunately, as a guy, I thought about it for a long time, and men are stupid. We just grunt at one another, we don't really talk, so I figured out "Look, I'll become a sportsman because there's only two phrases that men really use, which is "nice shot", "big fish", and the rest is just grunting." I became a sportsman because of that. That's how I socialized for all those years. But now, I'll talk to anybody. Any bum on the street, I'm yours, let's talk.

Chris: Do you regret that you waited that long to have one?

Richard: Absolutely. And you know what, it's not uncommon because I've been to meetings where the leader of the meeting will have 100 people in the room and he'll say, "Who regrets getting a cochlear implant?" And not a single arm will go up. And then he'll say, "Well who regrets not having it done sooner?" And a hundred hands go up right away. So yes, waiting is not really a great option. Sometimes you must wait for the technology to catch up with you, and right now the technology is spectacular. What the future brings, there's no way to predict. But I've kind of thought our time on earth is limited and to take advantage of it because you don't get a second chance. One around is all you get, and I finally woke up one day and said "Fine. This is great, this is what I'm doing."

Chris: What are the features you like best about the company that you chose and the model you chose?

Richard: Originally when I chose the N6, it was state of the art. The N7 pairs with an iPhone. I have my iPhone, if the phone rings, I click it, and the sound goes right to my processor. I listen to Intranet Radio on my iPhone. When you're listening to Intranet Radio on the iPhone, it's stereo.

They have other accessories called the Mini Mic, the TV Streamer, those will come in mono], but it sends the sound right to your head. Now, all the companies have accessory to help you do that. What I love about my Cochlear Mini Mic is if I go to a big dinner, there are 200 people in the room, I take the Mini Mic, put it on my table with 10 people sitting around, and the sound will come right to my processor. Which means I have the best hearing in the house. People are always turning to me saying "What did they say? What did they say?" I'm the deaf guy in the house, and they're asking me what's going on. This is kind of cool.

Chris: What kind of features would you like to see in the future for cochlear implants?

Richard: I've thought about this a lot. Guess what? I can't even foresee something better right now. I know that everybody gets a slightly different experience out of this because some people say the battery will them a day, the battery will last them nine hours. It's based on what we call the MAP. It's the programming, the individual programming. One thing I like to remind people, no two hearing losses are the same. They're all different, and no two solutions are the same. The Cochlear can modify and adjust to the individual, and that's what's very important to me.

Chris: How about music now?

Richard: That's why I'm here at Daddy O's record store. I was afraid in the beginning that it would sound mechanical. No question, the cochlear implants were developed for speech first. Music takes a little more time. But the reason I like to come back to a vinyl, I can differentiate the difference between the clear sound of a CD, and the warm sound of a vinyl. And that's just unbelievable to me. I started studying languages, I started studying Latin, and with my Cochlear I can differentiate the different sounds between a sound of b-u and p-u, I can hear the differences. What more could you ask for? So, I love coming here, I love collecting vinyl records again.

Chris: What are your favorite artists or groups?

Richard: Any jazz, I love jazz. Now, I must tell you when I first started listening to music my taste would change. Listening to the songs I remember from the 60s and 70s did not sound right. I had to develop a technique for rehabilitation, and I found that listening to YouTube videos, with the words, your brain and the music start to kick together. Some people take a year or more to hear music properly, I probably took six months. When you're rehabilitating, you have to work at it. There's no question, this is not a magic bullet, This is something that requires rehabilitation, but it's pleasurable.

Chris: Can you do it at home?

Richard: Yeah, oh yes. Matter of fact, of all the people I've mentored, a lot of people live alone, and I had to develop a rehabilitation system for them to work on their own, and it's fine. They get their hearing back.

Chris: You mentioned insurance. Do most people find that they'll be able to get coverage?

Richard: Most people do, even if you're on Medicare, because I've mentored people up to the age of 86 and they're on Medicare. Medicare will pay for one at a time, so even if you qualify for two you might have to go for your second one in six months or a year later, but that's part of it. Insurance companies cover by and large. Even if the insurance company says no, no does not mean no. One thing the Cochlear will do, they have a department that will fight for you.

Chris: What goals do you now have since you're able to hear?

Richard: (Laughing) I want to become a rock 'n' roll star.

Chris: Any advice for other people?

Richard: Don't wait. I'm telling you, if you're on the fence there are so many people who are out there to talk to about their experience, and I understand the fear. I understand the fear very, very well. But keep your eye on the prize of restored hearing, get out of isolation. I know you're in isolation from your family, from your friends, if you have problems with business, there's a solution for you. So, that's what I'd tell them.

Chris: Thank you very much.

CHAPTER 2 CHRIS GOODIER

HEARING LOSS ENDED HER CAREER

Growing up with normal hearing, Chris woke up one morning when she was 32, to discover she had lost her hearing in one ear. The sudden hearing loss was compounded by a progressive loss on the other side.

With no hearing on one side and a series of powerful hearing aid on the other, she struggled to keep her job. But one day, she realized the fight was futile. Her hearing was too far gone.

Being told by a succession of doctors that there was nothing they could do for her or that a cochlear implant was not the answer because the "sounded mechanical," she adapted a new vocation which allowed her to isolate herself.

Happily, she attended a convention of the Hearing Loss Association of America where she was able to collect brochures and information that led her to getting cochlear implant surgery and activated with a Cochlear Kanso processor.

Today she is bimodal, a ReSound Hearing aid on one side and a

Cochlear Kanso on the other. Fully functional she has joined the world of sound again.

Chris Goodier: I thought it was due to ear wax and ignored it, disregarded it, thought it would go away, but eventually, I went to see just

18

an MD who referred me to otolaryngologist, and they didn't know what had caused it, an unknown origin one-sided hearing loss. Eventually, when it continued to get worse and involved vertigo balance issues over time, I had a lot of tests where they suspected a brain tumor, any number of causes. Years later, it was diagnosed as autoimmune inner ear disease. By that time, I had almost no hearing in one ear, couldn't be helped by a hearing aid and was given a hearing aid for the other ear. That was more than 20 years ago. I've worn every type of hearing aid, completely in the canal, little, tiny ones. Now, I have the most powerful type over the ear in one ear, but I was still not hearing words. No speech comprehension because it was a progressive condition.

Chris Goodier: Some people with autoimmune inner ear disease lose all hearing overnight. Mine was gradual progressive to the point where I've had severe to profound loss in both ears. At that point, I finally had the nerve to have a cochlear implant. Now, I can hear very well out of that ear, and it get by with the other ear.

Richard: "Get by," meaning what?

Chris Goodier: Kind of-

Richard: Do you comprehend words in the other ear?

Chris Goodier: Yeah. The two work together very well. The ear with the hearing aid, now, is such a good hearing aid that I can make telephone calls with Bluetooth, much the same as the N7 Cochlear implant. I have Bluetooth capability-

Richard: Which one do you prefer when you're on the phone?

Chris Goodier: I have no Bluetooth with this ear because it's a Kanso processor.

Richard: Right.

Chris Goodier: I'm able to talk on the phone with this ear.

Richard: When you have the autoimmune disease, it was not stress related. In other word, did you-

Chris Goodier: It's hard to say. They don't really know, but it was diagnosed with a blood test.

Richard: Okay. You have a hearing loss. When you were in school you were functioning fine. Everything happened after you're out of school.

Chris Goodier: I was okay until that day when I was 32 years old. Just working-

Richard: Where are you working at the time?

Chris Goodier: Back in those days, I was in Washington, D.C. I was a sales marketing rep for a cruise line. I did that for numerous years. I worked for hotel chains. Mostly, in the cruise industry, travel agencies, doing sales and marketing work. That led to doing cruises for nonprofit groups. Most people are familiar with cruises, where your university or museum has a group and if fundraising office likes to have some of their top donors travel and bond with one another and with the organization. I began doing that type of cruise in Washington, D.C. for the National Symphony Orchestra, other organizations, the Kennedy Center for the Performing Arts. They were one of our best clients. They ultimately hired me to work in special events and fundraising.

Richard: Let me ask you a question. You noticed your hearing is gone or deteriorating. Talk to me a little bit about how it affected your career. Was there a particular day when you came to the realization you had a problem? That's what I'd like to know about.

Chris Goodier: When I was doing fundraising at the Kennedy Center, I had gotten a hearing aid. I was getting a lot okay. If I called on a client, I had to be sure that I could see their face. I realized, now, I was reading lips, learning unconsciously, but as I was promoted in the organization, I started overseeing major gifts, endowment, and plan giving donors. Major gifts are people who give the Kennedy Center $100,000 a year. It's important to hear every word they say because you're having lunch. When you have hearing loss in one ear, you're always trying to get the right chair on the right side so you can hear the person you're talking to. If he gets stuck with the deaf ear, you're going to have to keep turning and reading their lips, but I got by.

Chris Goodier: However, the Kennedy Center is an enormous, cavernous building. We began doing these small luncheons and dinner parties. When they were in rooms with the low ceiling, no problem. The carpeting, the acoustics were okay, but we started using spaces that had enormous ceilings. One night, I was sitting there, and I just realized I could not hear a word this man was saying even if I looked at him. Of course, there's somebody on the other side. I had to be able to talk to both people. Richard: How did you feel about it?

Chris Goodier: Panic, panic stricken. I really thought I cannot do this job anymore. I'm doomed. This was 20 years ago, and cochlear implants were not really in common use. My otolaryngologist office essentially said, "There's nothing we can do for you."

Richard: Did you investigate any devices that could compensate or overwork with-

Chris Goodier: No, because I had been told that the deaf ear, there was nothing. I only got by with one inadequate hearing aid at that point.

Richard: Can you talk about the telephone? How did you deal with the phone?

Chris Goodier: I only use the one ear with the hearing aid. Again, it was gradual and incremental. We had a pretty good phone system. I could understand people on the phone.

Richard: How long a period from the time you started losing the hearing to when the phone wouldn't work for you anymore?

Chris Goodier: Oh gosh, 20 years. Losing the phone really happened big time about 10 years ago. I just finally had to have my husband talk on the phone. What happened to my career is, really, that it was a very stressful environment. The goal setting was intense in any fundraising office. If it's any good, you are expected to produce X million dollars a year in gifts. I had my people, my targets. I found new donors. I was doing well, but then I would get in those situations that I described and that was scary. I had to just-

Richard: You had supervisors over you on, I'm sure. You have people over your-

Chris Goodier: Yeah. Yeah. Right.

Richard: How did they approach your hearing loss? What happened?

Chris Goodier: I think I was so good at faking it. That they weren't aware that I had such a severe loss because you compensate in so many ways. You don't get yourself into that kind of situation.

Richard: Talk a little bit more about compensation.

Chris Goodier: You try to always sit in the right place. You avoid certain situations. If you know that this a bad room or it's a huge crowd and you try to bluff your way through and say things like "Well, I'm sure everybody's having trouble today hearing in here, right?" People are like "Oh yeah, it's so hard in this crowd. I understand." Then you're like ... I've got a free pass to have to say, "Repeat that to me. What did you say?" Inside, you're like "Oh my gosh."

Richard: Well, your supervisor supports it because you're reaching your goal. Did you come to your own realization it was time to get out or did somebody come to you and say you're not?

22

Chris Goodier: Nobody ever came to me. It was me saying, "I can only keep faking for so long." Washington, D.C., that world ... the people we were dealing with were cabinet officials, famous writers, Alan Greenspan and his wife, Andrea Mitchell. These were the people who came to our dinner parties. I had a staff and I had them do a lot of the ... "I need you at the door to catch the name of the person who came in." Richard: That's confrontational.

Chris Goodier: Yeah, but there were also times where they weren't going to be allowed into an event. It was me standing there having to say to the chairman of the center, "Paul Newman is coming in." Now, I know who Paul Newman is. That was okay, but if it's someone who says, "I'm my own show." They're a mumbler. Boy, that's scary. Sometimes the chairman would be, "Oh, Fred, you're here." I would be, "Whew." I knew that the faking was only going to go so far for so long.

Richard: Have you seen people who have a hearing loss in your situation do a lot of faking like that?

Chris Goodier: Absolutely. Because nobody wants to be the one in the room with all the top managers in your department and say, "I have a hearing loss, so you guys are going to have to look at me and not all talk at once." Now, you can try that. There's nothing wrong with being upfront, but in a competitive environment, you don't want to be the guy who's the weak link. You don't want to be the one who must make other people change their mode just for you, so you don't ask. Or if you do and your friends understand, they work with you. They forget.

Richard: Talk about-

Chris Goodier: The meeting goes on.

Richard: Talk about your friends who were losing a hearing and talk about supportive. Were friends supportive of what was going on? Did anybody disappear and say, "I can't deal with this"?

Chris Goodier: I don't know. Maybe. What happened is, we decided to leave Washington and move to the Caribbean because my husband had been very ill. Luckily, he survived stage three cancer, but he thought, "Life is short. I'm going to retire young." I said, "I support you 100%. This is a stressful place. We'll get more money next year. In the year after, we'll both get more money in our jobs, but what does it matter if we don't have a quality life?" I was ready to check out of that stressful environment because hearing loss is stressful when you're covering and coping, but it's also exhausting to try and hear people.

Richard: Talk about how exhausting.

Chris Goodier: Yeah.

Richard: Talk about how.

Chris Goodier: Anybody who is struggling at work, in social events, family, you're always struggling to understand or to keep asking. I would joke with my husband and say, "You're talking to the refrigerator, I'm over here. You need to face me when you talk to me." You're always fighting to be able to understand. It is exhausting. You take naps if you can.

Richard: Yes. Now, your husband ... obviously, spouses are very important issue with people who have a hearing loss. Can you tell me a little bit about how he coped with it?

Chris Goodier: Well, he was terrific. He will always be a terrific person. In the last 10 years, before I got a cochlear implant and a better hearing aid, I would make him make all the phone calls. I can't talk on the phone. I always gave his phone number out. I had a cell phone number, but I only had it for emergencies. If I had to yell on the phone, "Our house is burning down. Come home." I didn't really get calls on that line or I would have to hand it to him.

Richard: Since you had your cochlear implant, do you still do that?

24

Chris Goodier: No.

Richard: You do your own.

Chris Goodier: No. The Bluetooth hearing aid that I have now is so far better than any hearing aid I've ever-

Richard: What hearing aid are you using now?

Chris Goodier: It's ReSound. It was a top of the line compatible with Cochlear America's products. If I were to use a TV streamer or a handheld Mini Mic, they work together.

Richard: They do work either.

Chris Goodier: Yes. My husband did the phone calls. He is just a person who ... I think looking back, he would say, "I don't think Chris Goodier got what you were saying," and help me get people to repeat things.

Richard: If you were in a very social environment in your work when you had the hearing loss, did that drift away a bit or did you find yourself isolating yourself a little more?

Chris Goodier: Yes, to some extent. When we moved to the

Caribbean, we realized that this was the island of Saint Croix. It was a very social environment. We joined the yacht club. We would go to these dinner parties. It's like Florida with the tile floors and the echoing of sound. However, a lot of socializing in the Caribbean is outside, outdoor restaurants. It's a lot easier to hear in that kind of environment. I made friends there. However, some of them were old, old friends who had moved there.

Chris Goodier: I had built in community and there were friends. They understood if I had to say, "I didn't get what you all were talking about. Go back and tell me who, who are we talking about?" They would stick with me, but it's very different to try and meet new people. They don't understand and you don't want to, again, be the one who says, "Oh, you have to help here if you want to be my friend." Again, I was compensating by reading lips. I realized that in my work and everything.

Richard: How long were you in the Caribbean?

Chris Goodier: I lived there about eight years.

Richard: Once you got your cochlear implant just a few years ago, did that change how you approach people?

Chris Goodier: Oh, yes. It's night and day.

Richard: Talk about that a bit.

Chris Goodier: Well, in the Caribbean, I started easing away from situations like work situations into working on my own, independently. I have been a writer, an editor working out of my home at my computer, doing everything by email and that is a real great compensation. Email is God's gift to deaf People. We moved back up from the Caribbean and I continued that work. I'd never made new friends, where we lived in North Carolina. We lived there seven years, eight years. I had one friend because I was isolating myself by my career choice. I had relatives there. I saw them, did not make friends. Then forward to getting a cochlear implant, which has only been not quite two years, now, I don't hesitate to talk to anybody. It's a whole new life. I'm like everybody else now. That's the bottom line.

Richard: Do you have any regrets about getting a cochlear implant?

Chris Goodier: Not really. I almost got one back in 2011 and then waited six years. Probably, I should've done it sooner, but on the other hand, when I moved to Sarasota, I had found the quality of the healthcare and the whole community of people, surgeons, audiologist who specialize in cochlear implant rehab, other people, the Hearing Loss Association. It's been such a strong support group.

26

Richard: Tell me a little bit why you hesitated because it's not an uncommon thing for people to hesitate. How about your experience?

Chris Goodier: Well, first, one of my ear doctors said to me, "Oh, you don't want a cochlear implant. It is very artificial and robotic hearing. That would only be your last resort." I believed this guy. He's an authority figure. Like "Oh, okay. Okay. Well, I'm losing my hearing every year, but that doesn't sound like an option." Then another in North Carolina, ear doctor, says, "I don't think a cochlear implant is something you need." I really dug my heels in. Meanwhile, I had gone to National HLAA conference and gathered all the material from the manufacturers. I was scared. I feared the surgery.

Chris Goodier: These two doctors saying, "No, no." That gave me the reason to procrastinate and convince myself, "Well, they must be right." Even though I've met all these people who said, "Oh, I wish I had never delayed." Then my big procrastination along with the fear was the misconception that, "Get it done and technology moves on and there you are. You're stuck with the 2011."

Richard: That didn't turn out to be true.

Chris Goodier: No. I had to go to a seminar where a Cochlear rep stood up there and brought home the point that, "The great thing here is, you have this little gadget, and we can reprogram that, and we can reprogram the device inside your inner ear, and you then get the benefit of the ongoing technology." That point had never reached me before.

Richard: Well, how did you make your choice for Cochlear?

Chris Goodier: That was hard. I had a friend who had one of the other manufacturers. Then I had a new friend here who had another one different. I didn't really know anybody who had a Cochlear brand implant, but I was convinced that they had the longest track record. The most people all over the world with that much success, thousands and thousands of people compared to much smaller numbers by the other two manufacturers. That gave me a confidence level.

Richard: You had single-sided deafness. Was there any discussion about the success of a single-sided deafness versus bilateral? What came up?

Chris Goodier: I talked to the surgeon about which ear he thought he would do. He felt the deaf ear was the one to go with, even though it had been 20 years since I had had any kind of good hearing out of that ear. He went with the worst one because I still have very borderline under Medicare. Medicare once below 40% speech comprehension in the best dated conditions in both ears and this year was borderline. The decision, really, was go with the worst one and that turned out to be the right decision.

Richard: Talk to me about music a little bit. What's your experience with it now?

Chris Goodier: Unlike a lot of people, music hasn't been a huge part of my world since the teenage years when you knew every single song, you knew every word. However, then, when I worked at the Kennedy Center, I would go and listen to the National Symphony Orchestra because I had free tickets anytime I wanted to go. I did a lot of their fundraising. I could go into an empty auditorium and sit there and hear Pavarotti rehearsing with National Symphony Orchestra. Just me and this rehearsal. Back then, music was important. The conductor was Rostropovich, world's greatest cellist when he was alive, really. I can remember just being riveted by his music. I think what happened is, when we left and went to the Caribbean, there were no performances. There were no concert halls. I stopped going to the movies because it was too hard to understand.

Chris Goodier: I didn't realize what was happening and that was that music had become very tinny. I still kind of got it, but it sounded off key, relay worked. I didn't really realize that, I guess, until we came back to the US. I just avoided music.

Richard: What about today?

Chris Goodier: It is coming back. One of the interesting things to me is that it's almost two years since I had my implant, but the curve continues to improve. One way I know this is that one of my favorite things was always to listen to CBS Sunday morning with the opening trumpet solo by Wynton Marsalis. It just sounded awful. I knew what it's supposed to sound like and that was not it. This sounded off key and weird. Did they just change octaves? What's going on here? Since I had my cochlear implant, it's kind of my little bellwether, my little checkpoint. On Sunday morning, I listened to that every week. It's now sounding normal. I'm getting my musical hearing back.

Richard: Travel now is better or worse. You can hear. Can you tell me a little bit about travel because I really love it?

Chris Goodier: Yeah. Really, one of the tipping points for getting a cochlear implant was, I went on a solo trip up to Kentucky to go to an alumni board meeting. Long story, but there was a blizzard. We're riding along on the airplane and there's an announcement. If you're hearing impaired, you hear that as [inaudible 00:24:57] Knoxville. You're like "Knoxville?" I'm looking around and asked this person because everyone is now grumping and like "Oh, no." They're pulling out their phones. I said, "What about Knoxville?" The woman said, "We're going to land there because there's a blizzard in Lexington and they don't know yet." When the flight attendant came by, I said, "I will need help because I cannot understand the overhead announcements, and in the airport, I'm going to need someone to tell me where to go." She said, "No problem. We will do that." They did not. It was the longest night of my life. Very, very difficult situation. Again, panic. I don't know if I think I recognize that person. I must chase them.

Chris Goodier: Then you fast forward to two months after I got a cochlear implant, a friend died. I decided to go to the funeral. My husband couldn't go. I went by myself, got on a plane to Dallas airport, no problem. Everybody is sitting down. I happened to be in a row that for some reason had to empty seats because the plane was full. The flight attendant comes down the aisle and leans over and whispers, "Would you be willing to move to first class? I need three seats together for a family." I said, "Yes." Now, a year before, (1) I wouldn't have been there by myself, but (2) I would have had to say, "What?" I don't want to say out loud, "Do you want to move to first class?" They would've said, "Never mind." They would've gone and found somebody else. I could hear the captain-

Richard: Let me ask you another question. Now, what is your greatest disappointment or regret? Do you have any since you got the cochlear implant?

Chris Goodier: No. Not one.

Richard: What's your goal for the future now that you can hear again?

Chris Goodier: Well, to do a good job on my book promotion tour.

Richard: Talk about your book.

Chris Goodier: Well, before I got a cochlear implant, I got a hearing dog from Dogs for Better Lives. I learned a lot about traveling with a service dog and became friends with a deaf author named Henry Kaiser. He had a service dog. He wanted to go on a cruise. I said, "I can tell you all about it. It's complicated, paperwork involved." Together, we shared our information. Henry is a train buff and between the knowledge base we both had about traveling with these dogs, we realized there's no resource. You just must try and find people who can tell you what you're supposed to do about it if you want to export your dog from the United States on a trip.

Chris Goodier: We agreed to write a book. We pitched it to the University of Illinois press and they accepted it and it's coming out in September 2019.

Richard: The title is?

Chris Goodier: Traveling with Service Animals.

Richard: That's very exciting.

Chris Goodier: It is. It helps greatly that I can hear because I could be interviewed. I could be on television if I need to. I can go talk to anyone on the telephone who has questions if they're writing about the book. That's my goal right now, to promote that.

Richard: Do you have any advice for others?

Chris Goodier: For people who have hearing loss?

Richard: Yes.

Chris Goodier: I guess just do something about it. Don't stay home and isolate yourself. It's going to cut your life short. It could lead to Alzheimer's disease. You got to stop that thinking, get the best hearing aid you can possibly afford. Then if that's not doing the job, get evaluated for cochlear implant. Technology can be a miracle in your life. It was in mine.

Richard: Terrific.

CHAPTER 3 DAVID DORSEY

A HYBRID COCHLEAR IMPLANT RECIPIENT

David Dorsey's high frequency hearing loss was interfering with his job as a reporter and was a strain on him and his family.

He was a thorough researcher. He wanted to retain whatever natural hearing he had. In his case a hybrid cochlear implant was the best possible solution. A hybrid cochlear implant is a combination of a cochlear implant with a hearing aid component. David's search led him far afield from home until he found a surgeon in which he had full confidence.

His high frequency hearing loss probably started when he was very young. Like many others, he did not realize he had a problem until he was an adult, and his story speaks to many of us who lived in denial of our hearing loss.

Happily, he received an Advanced Bionics hybrid, and he talks about his progress and the changes it brought to his life.

NOTE: David Dorsey became a bilateral cochlear implant recipient in 2021

Richard: Talk a little bit about your hearing loss. How did you lose your hearing loss?

David Dorsey: Well, I think I was just born and that's how I lost it. It depends on which doctor I'm talking to. Some of the doctor's think I was born without high-frequency hearing, and some of the doctor's think that maybe I was four or five and maybe I took an antibiotic that was over-toxic and bad for my hair cells in the inner ear. But it doesn't really matter. I mean, I couldn't hear high frequency for the bulk, if not all of my life. So, talking about the top keys on a piano. I'm talking about when you hit a microwave button, the beeping or in my car, I've got a Subaru and they have a lot of warning sounds in the car. Like if there's a car in your blind spot, and the warning alarm goes, "Bing!" I couldn't hear that before I got the implant.

Richard: Did you have any siblings with hearing problems? Brothers or sisters with a hearing problem?

David Dorsey: No. They're fine. I have three brothers, and they all can hear much better than I can.

Richard: How long did you wear hearing aids? When did you lose your hearing?

David Dorsey: I think I knew in high school. I was always shy because I didn't like being around big groups of people talking. So, I tended to do better in one-on-one friendships, and not big groups hanging out talking together. That put me at a disadvantage in high school. You know, when you're in high school everyone's kind of hanging out together, and I would prefer to talk with a friend by himself because when you get a lot of voices, I just couldn't function really well.

Richard: Were you wearing hearing aids back in high school?

David Dorsey: I didn't know that I was deaf. It wasn't really until college, when I was 20, 21, when I really started to go see an audiologist and where they'd be like, "Hey, you're deaf." Or not, "You're deaf," but "You can't hear high frequency." I did not get a hearing aid until much, much later. I'm 47 now and I was maybe 32 when I got the hearing aid.

Richard: So, it was a long time. When you were in college, did you have any coping mechanisms to get through school?

David Dorsey: No. I did fine. For the most part, I was in a small classroom. I went to the University of Kansas, which was a big, giant school but for the most part, I took classes in small classroom environments. So, I would only have 10 or 15 kids in most of my classes. The classes where I had the big, arena style classes, I just got through it. I'm no genius but I think I got a 3.0 GPA, which is good enough and I had healthy B average.

Richard: How did you deal with the big classroom? What did you do in college when you were in a big classroom, and it was difficult to hear? That's what I'm trying to find out. Did you have a coping mechanism in particular classroom?

David Dorsey: I would always sit as close as I could in all my classes. I have always been one to sit at the front of the class. Like I said, I think I was in denial. I know I was in denial for a long time about having hearing loss. I didn't want to have anything wrong with me. Nobody likes to have anything wrong with them. So, it really wasn't until I decided to get the implant, where I was kind of like, all in on needing one, you know, "I can get through. I can do this." That's kind of always the attitude that I've had. That's good and healthy except for when you're in denial about being able to get something done and you think you can do it and you really can't. That's a problem.

David Dorsey: For many years, I was a sportswriter here at The News Press and one of my responsibilities in my mid-to-late 20s was taking high school sports results phone call and I didn't have the hearing aids for a lot of those years. I butchered a lot of names. I wish I could apologize to every teenager that I misspelled their name.

Richard: Can you talk about one specific incident?

David Dorsey: I don't remember anything real specific, but I can tell you that the consonants in human speech, most consonants fall in the frequency I can't hear. So, the S's and the F's and the PH's and the Z's, they all kind of jumble together for me. Even now that I have the implant, it's not perfect and I'm on the phone just yesterday and we're talking about a real estate development deal, what's going to be built on this corner and he said, "Keke's Breakfast Café," but it took me like three or four or five times to get the word right. Because it's, you know, Keke's is K-E-K-E, but my brain wasn't figuring out what he said.

David Dorsey: After the implant it takes some time to adapt to this.

Richard: How long have you had the implants now?

David Dorsey: I had the surgery on December 7th, and I had the activation on January 11th. Most people wait a month. I waited five weeks because I got it done at the University of Iowa. I wanted to wait an extra week and wait to heal.

Richard: We'll come back to that in a little while because I have more questions about your vocation and your job.

David Dorsey: Okay.

Richard: Were there particular support that you had at your job here? Once you knew you had a severe hearing loss, did your fellow employees here, were they supportive or did you have problems?

David Dorsey: Yes. Yes. The News Press has been tremendously supportive. When I did get the hearing aids, they were a game changer for me. They helped a lot. Not as much the implant but they helped a lot. Especially Phonak, they make a device called the Com Pilot and that was a game changer for me because when you get a Com Pilot, it funnels the voice into your hearing aid or your implant. I still use the same Com Pilot that

I've had for a long time. When I answer the phone, I just hit a button and the voice goes right into my devices.

Richard: Do you have to hold the phone in front of you at that point?

David Dorsey: At one point I did have a device that was compatible with the Com Pilot that I could hook-up to my work phone. I used that for a while. Then I found that just dealing with my cellphone was better for me and more convenient. While most of my colleagues have a cellphone and a work phone, I talked to my bosses and I said, "You know what, I don't want the work phone anymore. I just want to do everything off my cell."

Richard: It's not an uncommon situation you're talking about where people work in an office and there's an office phone and they have their cell. So, that's why I'm trying to find out from you how you dealt with it because other people want to know.

David Dorsey: Yeah. I did have a colleague in a different department that she just had a caption phone where when someone speaks, it will transcribe what they say. I think it's called a CapTel phone, right? I've never had one of those. I have heard that there's a delay and, in my vocation, it's just better for me to hear. You mentioned a coping mechanism, with being a reporter with a hearing deficit, it's a dangerous combination. Not the best thing.

David Dorsey: So, couple things I'll do is, if I am in a crowded environment, I'll pull the guy aside, or woman, aside and go, "Hey, listen. I don't hear well. Can we step into a quiet area?" I've done that a lot.

Richard: How do people react?

David Dorsey: They're like, "Hey, yeah. Sure, no problem," but I can't even think of a time where someone looked at me funny. You must have a little bit of confidence though and know your limitation. The other thing that I'll do, this happened a lot in what I call, "The dark time," which is the time between my implant surgery and the time of activation. I had a tough time hearing those five weeks. There were a lot of phone calls that I had to make to take care of stuff through the insurance company.

Richard: Did people make the phone calls for you when you couldn't hear [crosstalk 00:11:05].

David Dorsey: I did a lot of them. I did a lot of the calls. I'm only doing them through my hearing aid ear and not through this ear. This ear, my good ear, it qualifies for an implant as well.

Richard: How do you feel about that? Doing a second implant?

David Dorsey: I am so glad I did this one. At the time, I would've done both, had insurance allowed it. My insurance company will only allow one cochlear implant at a time. So, I chose to implant my left ear, which is worse than my right ear. Similar, but worse. The doctor recommended I do the worse ear first. They told me that-

Richard: Did you have any input into which ear to do?

David Dorsey: Yeah, it was my choice. I wanted to get the worse ear done first. It just made sense to me because I do have a significant amount of hearing left in both ears now, but I had more hearing left in my right ear, and I didn't want to risk losing it through the surgery.

Richard: Talk a little bit about residual hearing and fear of losing it. That's a very, very common issue for people who are candidates for cochlear implants. Their fear of losing residual hearing. Talk about your feelings of that.

David Dorsey: So, it's a healthy fear to have, to not want to lose the hearing that you have, to get back with the implant. I'll be honest with you; it probably took me an extra two to three years to get the implant done because of that fear. In 2003, Dr. Luetje in Kansas City, he was very renowned, and he is retired now, but he is one of the pioneers in cochlear implants. He wrote me a letter, looking at my audiograms, and he said... This is in 2003. He said, "I want you to wait for two things to happen before you get your implant. I want you to wait for your hearing to get worse," because at the time the hybrids weren't a thing yet. They usually just knock out all your natural hearing and not think about your residual hearing. Then he said, "The second thing I want you to do, is I want you to wait for us to get better. I want you to wait for the technology to get better."

David Dorsey: So, in 2018, I decided that well, my hearing got worse, and the technology got better. So, I followed his advice 15 years later.

Richard: No regrets?

David Dorsey: No regrets. Even though I'm so glad that I got this left ear done. I'm also glad that they didn't let me do the right ear because of the whole music situation. I like listening to music and with the implant, I've been told that it takes a good year to adapt to music. Now I'm four months into this, I really got another eight months to get to maybe where I'm going to be, music is kind of blurry. Okay. Like, human speech is getting so much better. Cochlear implants were designed with that in mind. They were designed with understanding human speech better. They weren't designed so much as to help you listen to a symphony orchestra better.

David Dorsey: I'm finding that if I listen to one instrument at a time, it comes in better than if I'm hearing the whole band. I've also found that my good ear, if you will, sometimes helps my implanted ear in understanding things, especially with music. However, my implanted ear helps my good ear a lot, especially with consonant sounds in speech but in music with all these sounds that I can't hear with this ear at all, percussion, drums, cymbal, the tambourine, the keyboard, and a piano. So, the terms are bilateral, which is what you are when you have two implants or two hearing aid, or bimodal, which is what I am now, where I've got an implant and a hearing aid.

David Dorsey: So, the surgeon was like, "Well, in six months you might start thinking about wanting the second one," but I'm not there yet.

Richard: But you also have something that's unusual, which is a hybrid cochlear implant, and it's not that common, right? It's not- David Dorsey: No, it's not that common.

Richard: Why did you decide on the hybrid?

David Dorsey: Actually, the doctor and some of the companies are trying to get away from the hybrid term now because they're really trying to mainstream hearing preservation in the patients now. My surgeon, it was a big thing with him, and he's done a lot of these surgeries. He's done more than 300 hybrids, if you will and that was why I went to Iowa because I had a comfort level with his experience. His name is Dr. Bruce Gantz. Since 1995, he's received more than 60 million dollars in grant money to research hearing preservation techniques.

David Dorsey: One of my hard-of-hearing colleagues said she wants to wait until they have stem cell hair regeneration. I told my doctor that, and he said, "Well, she's going to be waiting in a box, because that's not happening any time soon because it's science fiction right now that we can regenerate hair cells through stem cell techniques."

David Dorsey: Now, the next thing is going to be robots, okay? Because my surgeon's telling me that he's confident that a robot can insert the electrode into cochlear more efficiently than the human hand can and that there will be less chance of disrupting the healthy hair cells that are in there right now. I did not want to wait until the robots were ready. I was ready to become a robot myself at this time.

Richard: So, do you have no regrets about having…

David Dorsey: No regrets whatsoever, at all. I don't know how the future will unfold, nobody does. I can't tell you right now if I'm going to get this ear implanted also. Right now, I don't want it done but I'm not going to say I'm never going to get it done because this was so successful and helpful. However, there's certain things that I can do with this ear, that I can't with this.

Richard: Name one.

David Dorsey: The music is the biggest thing. Also, there are times when I can take off the hearing aid and the processor of the implant, I'd just take a walk around the block, right? I can still hear enough to get by because I have the residual hearing. Sitting here today, there's always a risk of losing the residual hearing through the surgery, and I've done it with this ear, and I'm fine with it. I did lose some residual hearing with this ear. I still have enough left to get by in an emergency type of situation.

David Dorsey: Not being able to hear, it's not the end of the world for me. Sometimes I enjoy my quiet moments.

Richard: Talk about the moments of quiet. When do you like quiet?

David Dorsey: Well, this morning I went swimming, okay? I'm not wearing my implant. Some people will get the waterproof case for their implant, but I haven't invested in that. But if I am swimming laps or if I'm out bike riding. When I'm out bike riding, I can't hear all the birds that I can hear with this thing.

Richard: So, talk about that. Yes. You can hear birds now, but you weren't able to before.

David Dorsey: Yeah, I mean who knew that so many birds made so much noise. I had no idea.

Richard: What about sounds around the house? What do you hear?

David Dorsey: Sounds around the house. The microwave, the oven. Like setting the oven timer, I could never hear the beeping on that before. One thing that hasn't changed is my dog. When he barks, and he barks incessantly sometimes, and I'm wondering if there's a way to program the implant to not pick up my dog barking, would be a wonderful programming thing, if they could find it all-

Richard: I want to ask you about your family. How do they deal with your hearing loss and when you decided to get a cochlear implant, were they supportive? Were they afraid? How did your family feel?

David Dorsey: My family was tremendously supportive. My wife was overjoyed because now I can hear her better. Now I don't have any excuses for... You know, we know the difference between hearing and listening, right? So, now that I can hear, I should be able to listen better, right? You know what, I can hear her better and it's tremendous.

Richard: What about your children?

David Dorsey: So, my son is 11. With him, because he's my son, we get it. He understands where I'm at with my hearing. It's more like when he's around with all his friend, so now I can understand better than I used to.

Richard: Now you spoke about the fact you waited, you kept delaying getting this done. Can you talk about who was the most important influence, what influenced you the most to decide to make the plunge?

David Dorsey: Well, you were a tremendous influence, believe it or not.

Richard: Why?

David Dorsey: Because-

Richard: That's flattering but there must have been other people out there.

David Dorsey: Well, yeah but it's you and there've been a couple other recipient besides yourself. There were three of you. One of them I met on Twitter. I've never met him in person, but he had both of his ears implanted. The company put me in touch with another guy that had both of his ears implanted. So, you have all this fear, it's helpful to talk to people who have been down that road before.

Richard: You know what I would love to know a little bit more about how you made your decision to, you know for the company you chose. What was there about the company that you decided to use that?

David Dorsey: I chose Advanced Bionics, partially because the surgeon had a good comfort level with the company. He inserts MED-EL and Cochlear as well, but he has a software program during the surgery that he told me only works with the Advanced Bionics brand. During the surgery he's able to monitor my existing hair cells and he was able to stimulate them and see them firing off. So, if he gets too close to them, he was able to back off in sort of the electrode around the sensitive areas. I'm not into this whole brand snobbery. I can't tell anyone that my brand of implant is better than your brand or this other guy's brand. But guess what, I can't try all three and then decide.

David Dorsey: It really shouldn't matter. All three companies are great, and all three are going to help you hear better.

Richard: But the surgeon was the one who...

David Dorsey: I think all the surgeons develop relationships with the different companies. So, if you talk-

Richard: Have you been traveling since you got your implant?

David Dorsey: You know what? I've only flown once since I've gotten it, but there's not trouble like at the airport or anything like that.

Richard: Can you hear the announcements now?

David Dorsey: I don't know because I've only done one flight. So, I'm going to take a trip later this summer, and I'll pay better attention because you got to remember the first five weeks after activation were a big challenge because my brain was just trying to figure out what all these noises meant. So, I think I would understand the announcements better now than I did.

Richard: Now that you have an implant, can you accomplish something you haven't done before? Or having goals in the future now that you have your implant?

David Dorsey: Gosh, it's been four months. So, career-wise I seem to be trending upward. I have a new newspaper column that runs every Tuesdays on news-press.com. I don't know. I can't sit here and tell you that if I hadn't had the surgery, they wouldn't have given me the column, but maybe when I got back and they realized I was hearing better, they were-

Richard: Do you have any advice for other people who are considering?

David Dorsey: For people on the fence you mean, right?

Richard: Yes.

David Dorsey: Yeah. So, if you're on the fence, I'm not here to give anybody medical advice but I would encourage anyone on the fence to do as much research as you can. Look at all three companies. Research the doctors and find out from them. Ask them, "Hey, how many of these surgeries have you done?" I ended up traveling to Iowa to get mine done. I'm not saying someone on the fence has to go to Iowa and see Dr. Gantz. But these surgeries are starting to increase. We got a large portion of the population getting older and losing their hearing and more doctors are learning the techniques. So, I think there's more option now than ever before, but you got to be relentless in your research and don't just take what I say as the be all, end all. You want to find out for yourself who's the nearest doctor and who's the nearest, most experienced doctor.

Richard: I want to thank you for your time.

David Dorsey: I really appreciate you coming down here and spreading the message of the cochlear implant.

Richard: Thank you so much for your time.

David Dorsey: All right. Thanks.

Chapter 4 Maria Anderson

Running Towards Hearing Again

Maria Anderson is a shining example of a cochlear implant recipient who has never let them slow her down for a moment.

A marathon runner, hiker, and adventurer she recently completed a marathon in Greenland while wearing her Advanced Bionics processor clipped to her running shorts. She has also hiked Kilimanjaro, and to the base camp of Mt. Everest as well as around Mount Blanc.

Maria's hearing loss began in her mid-30s. She continued to compensate, determined not to wear a hearing aid so not to show her disability. She continued to struggle for 10 years before a total loss in her right ear forced her to reconsider.

She received an Advanced Bionics implant in 2007 and two years later went bilateral. Both operations were done by Dr. John Niparko at Johns Hopkins.

She discusses her fear of losing the 8% residual hearing in her left before going bilateral, her work environment, and the support from her family.

At first embarrassed by her deafness, she discovered the Sarasota chapter of the Hearing Loss Association of America where she learned how to advocate for herself, and others and her insights are invaluable and mentoring to help others has become a passion.

Richard: It's not easy to catch Maria. A runner, a traveler, and an adventurer. It took three tries to get her to sit down and talk about her hearing journey. And her lifestyle choices that helped her select her Advanced Bionics cochlear implant and processors. Diagnosed with a hearing loss in her mid-thirties, by her own admission she was too vain to wear hearing aids. And as her hearing declined, she was forced to reconsider. She talks of her embarrassment of being deaf, and her journey to become an advocate for herself and others, after joining the Sarasota Chapter of the Hearing Loss Association of America. I was grateful for the 25 minutes she would spare me before she was off and running again.

Maria Anderson: What happened was that in my mid-thirties, I started to lose the ability to discriminate consonant. And what specifically happened is, I was sitting in a meeting, in a client meeting, and my colleague sitting next to me whispered a question to me. Richard, to this day, I have no idea what my colleague asked of me, because I just could not hear a darn thing. So I went to an ENT, and he had his audiologist test me. And they found that I needed to wear hearing aids in both ears. Well, here I am in my mid-thirties, and there was just no way that I was going to wear hearing aids. I was just too vain.

Richard: Was it a vanity issue? Okay.

Maria Anderson: Exactly.

Richard: Fine, okay.

Maria Anderson: I admit it. No way was I going to. I continued to compensate and my family, they were my accomplices and my compensation, as you know, until seven years later. No, about 10 years later,

46

excuse me, I lost hearing completely in my right ear. Could not hear anything at all. Went back to the ENT, he thought that it had been a viral infection, never mentioned getting a cochlear implant, and basically just encouraged me to get a hearing aid in the other ear.

Richard: And this was how long ago?

Maria Anderson: Let me see. It would have been probably around the year, 2000.

Richard: So almost 20 years ago?

Maria Anderson: Right, exactly, that this happened. I went ahead and I got a hearing aid in my left ear. And I worked, we socialize, life went on. Until the day I woke up, which was about seven years later, and I had 10% hearing left.

Richard: In one ear or both?

Maria Anderson: In the other ear.

Richard: Okay.

Maria Anderson: So, at that point I was forced to get a CI. And I went ahead and got it on my right ear, which was the first ear that I lost hearing in. And that was in the year 2007.

Richard: Okay.

Maria Anderson: Two years later I became bilateral and got my second CI.

Richard: I'd like to know why you decided to go bilateral, because that's a point that many, many candidates are thinking about.

Maria Anderson: Well, at that point, my hearing was continuing to deteriorate. It was really a question of time. I had already gone from the 10% that I had to 8% hearing. And the audiologist that I was seeing told me it's only going to get worse, Maria. One thing that he said to me that just sealed the deal for me was, he said, "Don't think about what you're going to lose. Think about what you're going to gain."

Richard: Were you afraid of losing the residual hearing?

Maria Anderson: Yes. I was so afraid of losing my residual hearing, I was so afraid of just being deaf.

Richard: If the residual hearing was only about 8% at that time, and you still had the fear?

Maria Anderson: Exactly. And I know today that does not sound logical, but it really was a major step for me to say, "Okay, I need to look at what I'm going to gain." And it was amazing Richard, to see how much I had been missing, once I got that second CI. It was eye-opening. And I realized again, how noisy the world can be.

Richard: I want to go back one second, because obviously you lost your hearing after college, after high school, way later.

Maria Anderson: Exactly.

Richard: What were you doing for work? What was your career?

Maria Anderson: I worked for a pharmacy benefit manager, and I was in customer service operations. I was the face of member services for one of our larger clients. I had a lot of client meetings, lots of conference calls. I mean that's what my day was about at work.

Richard: Did you leave that job, or you stayed with it?

Maria Anderson: No, after I got my CIs, I was back at work, and I worked for five years until I retired. My hearing was never a performance issue.

Richard: That's very interesting, because a lot of people, when they have problems in high school or college, so on and so forth, and I've interviewed many like that. I've interviewed one before, who had a very good job in public relations, and she was forced to leave the job because of the hearing. But you never left the job?

Maria Anderson: I left the job for a reason that had nothing to do with my hearing loss.

Richard: And your hearing loss came after ADA was passed. Did that have any effect on you at all?

Maria Anderson: You know what, shame on me, Richard, because I did not use ADA at work. And I really should have asked for accommodations, but I was still at that point where I was not advocating for myself. I was still, I would almost say embarrassed by the fact that I had lost my hearing. I didn't want to be singled out at work as being different. You go with the flow. Were my days easy at work? No, not always, but I'll tell you, I had colleagues that just embraced my situation, and helped me so much at work. Especially when I first came back after my first cochlear implant.

Richard: Did everybody expect her to hear right away when you got it?

Maria Anderson: Yes, of course they did. But I made it known that I couldn't. I could attend small group meetings, but the conference calls, when you have 10 or 15 people on them with accents. And the speech, it's very rapid and the questions and the answers are flowing very quickly. That is what proved to be the most trying. And again, I was very fortunate that my colleagues supported me to the point that they would lend me their notes, they would send me instant messages to make sure that I grasp a certain decision that they knew was key to me. Things like that. No, I was blessed.

Richard: You were absolutely blessed, because that's very, very rare that that happens.

Maria Anderson: Exactly.

Richard: But you said something very interesting to me. I'd like to know, when did you start advocating for yourself?

Maria Anderson: After I retired and joined HLAA. I must give the Sarasota/Manatee Chapter full credit for that. It was by attending their meetings Richard, that I've came to understand that I had to advocate for myself. Because if I don't tell you that I have hearing loss, how can I expect anyone else to tell you that I have hearing loss. Or for you to be able to help me in a situation. So again, it's getting over that, I don't want to stand out. I don't want to be different. But you know what? At one point, it just comes to the fact that we should not be embarrassed about our hearing loss.

Richard: What about your family, your family supported you fully, church?

Maria Anderson: Completely.

Richard: Everybody?

Maria Anderson: My husband Richard, from the day he heard that I needed hearing aids, to today has never blinked. He has stood by my side and supported me completely. My daughter knows when she comes to visit, she's got to get my attention first. Otherwise, Mom might miss what she's trying to say. Even one of my sisters, when we go out, will advocate for me, and she'll tell people, "You need to face her, because she has hearing loss." And I think it's wonderful. Now I'll tell you that when my family gets together, we are Cuban, and when we get together for the holidays, for reunions, just like Italians and Greeks, the conversation starts flowing, 40 people talking at once. And yes, I do get lost in some of those conversations, but it's funny because somebody will always say, "Hey, don't forget, she's not listening. She's not cuing in. We've lost her, basically. We've lost Maria."

Richard: You are blessed, no question. I'm going to ask you the other side of the coin. Who disappointed you when you lost your hearing?

Maria Anderson: I can only remember one situation that happened. I took my Volkswagen in to be serviced, and I could not understand the gentlemen, the service man that was going to take my car. And I told him that I had hearing loss, and he became very angry with me. And to this day I still don't understand why, but it was obvious in his tone of voice, the way he looked at me. Suddenly his speech got very loud, and I said, "You don't need to yell at me. Just look at me and please slow down." He had a heavy accent, and I didn't even bring that into the conversation. I just said, "Can you look at me when we're speaking." And I remember just being rattled.

Richard: Who advocated the most for you to get a cochlear implant, and how did you make your decision that day to do it?

Maria Anderson: Well, once again, when you have no hearing in one ear, and you wake up one morning and all you have is 10% in another, your options are very limited at that point. It was a decision that my husband and I made, that if I was going to function in a hearing world, I needed to get a cochlear implant. And Richard, I wanted it. I wanted to be able to communicate with my family, to socialize, to travel, to go to work, to be able to live my life again. We almost must stop seeing hearing loss, as this is the end of our world of our life. Rather it's just a little step that maybe we need to take to the side, but then we get right back on course. And that's what I wanted to do.

Richard: Did you have concerns about surgery?

Maria Anderson: I had my surgery done at Johns Hopkins. I went up there for a second opinion, because once again, when I lost my hearing completely, really, we didn't know anything about hearing loss. I saw a specialist in Tampa, who said I needed a CI. But then my husband went ahead and emailed Johns Hopkins for a consultation, and we went up there and met with one of their audiologists. And since we had traveled from Tampa, they also introduced me to Dr. John Niparko, who was the head of the listening center, and who ended up being my surgeon. In one visit I went ahead and got my answers about the CI and heard about the surgical procedure. I decided to go ahead and have the surgery done up at Johns Hopkins.

Richard: It's not uncommon that some of the candidates I've interviewed have traveled long distances for the second opinion. And you're reinforcing that to people who are doing research, you don't have to accept the first diagnosis. You can keep going and keep searching even if you must go far afield.

Maria Anderson: Exactly, and for me it was well worth the trip. The surgery for the most part, I was comfortable going into it, again because I had Dr. John Niparko doing it. Like anyone going through CI surgery, I think our biggest question is, will it be successful? Will I be able to hear? So yes, I went into it with those fears. And on activation day, I was able to hear words.

Richard: Wow.

Maria Anderson: My daughter and my husband accompanied me. And it's funny because my daughter's tone of voice just fits beautifully in my sweet spot. I was able to hear Christina better than I could, my husband. And even to this day. But I was able to hear some words when I was first activated. I returned to Johns Hopkins for the second CI as well. In fact, I used to travel to see my audiologist at Johns Hopkins.

Richard: Were you living in Florida at the time?

Maria Anderson: Yes. I would take a day off work, and I would fly up to Baltimore, meet with my audiologist, have the mapping done. And this went on for three years until Ryan left and went to work for Cochlear in Australia.

Richard: That's the next question. People want to know how to choose the brand. And if you know my website, it's nonspecific. And I'd be curious about how you went about choosing what you're wearing by the way, we haven't discussed that.

Maria Anderson: Okay. I wear Advanced Bionics Naida Q90. And we did a lot of research into the three brands. But the thing that I liked the most about AB, is the fact that they always seem to be a forerunner in technology. They're always pushing the edge of the envelope as far as technology is concerned, with features and all of that. The second thing that attracted me to Advanced Bionics, is their customer service. I wanted to know that if I had an issue with any aspect of the processor, or any part, whatever, that they would be responsive. And to this day I can tell you that I have not had any issue in the last 12 years with customer service.

Richard: What aspect of the Advanced Bionics do you like the best? You said there were features you like. What do you like the best of it?

Maria Anderson: What I like right now about the Naída Q90 is that it has five programs. I'm able to have one for telecoil. I also have one just for like regular conversations like you and I are having. I have a noise reducing program as well. I have a variety of features available basically at my fingertips.

Richard: Do you have any regrets?

Maria Anderson: Not even one. No, not at all Richard. Not a single regret that I chose Advanced Bionics. Not a single regret that I went bilateral. Not a single regret that I got my first implant. Like I said to you, what was most important to me is to continue to live my life, to be able to be as active as I always have been, and not to be a burden to anyone because of my hearing loss.

Richard: Your independence is the most important?

Maria Anderson: Yes, and that's a very good way of putting it. Absolutely.

Richard: Do you have any hobbies or travel, things you like to do that are better because of your cochlear implant?

Maria Anderson: As a matter of fact, and I think you know that I'm very much into running. Two and a half weeks ago, I ran a marathon in Greenland.

Richard: My gosh!

Maria Anderson: I know.

Richard: Wearing your cochlear implant?

Maria Anderson: Absolutely. Yes.

Richard: You never take it off?

Maria Anderson: In fact, I have summited Mount Kilimanjaro. I have hiked to base camp at Mount Everest. I have hiked around Mont Blanc, and all of this is of course wearing my CI. I have a Neptune, which is Advanced Bionics' version of a waterproof. That's their waterproof-
Richard: How does that work for you? Describe that a bit.

Maria Anderson: The processor, what I do is that I wear a long cable from my headpiece, all the way down to my running shorts. And I put the processor behind me so that I can control the volume. And because of the heat and humidity primarily here in Florida, I wear the Neptune. But anytime that I am physically active, that is the processor that I wear. I don't wear the behind the ear like the one that you and I are wearing right now.

Richard: Okay. And so that helps with running or swimming or-

Maria Anderson: Exactly. So that has allowed me to do one of my passions, which is running. Exactly.

Richard: What are you running away from?

Maria Anderson: No! (Laughing) We're running to.

Richard: Okay.

Maria Anderson: Look at it that way. And usually, it's a glass of wine at the end of the day.

Richard: All right now you have your hearing, I understand from you that you also mentor people who have Advanced Bionics. Can you talk a little bit about what you do when you mentor them?

Maria Anderson: Advanced Bionics has a meet-and-greet every month. And several of us that are mentors will come there, and we will then talk to folks that are considering getting a CI. Also, those who have recently become implanted, that have questions about the journey. And the thing is, I think what we see is that there is a common thread, that all of us share the same questions, the same fears. And you want to hear from somebody that's been through the process. And that especially has been successfully through the process, how it is, what it is that they did to help them get basically to the other side.

Richard: That's a very, very important point, because I probably spend 30 to 40 hours a week on Facebook. And we know that Facebook has a lot of bashing the other brand kind of thing. My brand is better than your brand. It's important for people to understand that even though these interviews are long, they're in depth. And that if you're really doing serious research, you need more than a five second answer. Take your time to research and you'll figure it out.

Maria Anderson: And, what's good about these meet-and-greets is, there's a couple of mentors there, so you learn different ways of handling the same situation. Also, if you have a question, you can then come back the following month if you want. We're also available by email. I do a lot of email mentoring, where people are not ready to get on the phone or anything, and they prefer the written word. And that's fine.

Richard: Are the meet-and-greet, different from HLAA meetings like this?

Maria Anderson: Yes.

Richard: Can you describe some of the differences?

Maria Anderson: Well, the meet-and-greet is Advanced Bionics specific, and it is done at the Tampa Hearing and Balance Center, in one of their conference rooms. Basically, what we talk about is the brand that we're wearing, and what a cochlear implant is and basically answer the questions of the people that are gathered there. HLAA on the other hand, basically provides information and support to those of us who have hearing loss. It can be anyone who wears a hearing aid, or someone who wears a hearing aid and a CI, whatever. It's I think probably a more of an umbrella type group, a very supportive group.

Richard: Let me ask you one last question. What would you like to tell people who are sitting on the fence?

Maria Anderson: Do it. You don't realize what you're missing until you go through it. Until you get your CI, and you see, and you hear all those little sounds that you haven't heard for years. It's a hard thing not to be afraid, but sometimes you just must take that step, and believe that you will come through it with flying colors. There is no reason why you won't.

Richard: Well, I thank you very, very much for your time.

Maria Anderson: You're welcome, Richard. I enjoyed it.

CHAPTER 5 LOU FERRIGNO

THE INCREDIBLE HEARING JOURNEY OF THE INCREDIBLE HULK

Champions are a breed apart. Their motivation and their dedication are far beyond average. Mohammed Ali said it best; "I hated every minute of training. But I said… Don't quit. Suffer now and live the rest of your life as a champion."

When the opportunity came to interview a recent cochlear implant recipient who also is a special champion I jumped at the chance. Lou Ferrigno at age twenty-one was the youngest Mr. Universe and later went on to win it two years in a row along with a long string of other wins in body-building competitions. His career included his best-recognized performance as The Incredible Hulk in the television series from 19771982.

In a recently published interview, Lou mentioned being bullied as a child for his hearing loss. I could identify with that. We both lost our hearing at about the same age and used analog body-worn hearing aids with a wire running to an earpiece. I was a skinny weakling, but I could not image anyone picking on Lou and live to tell the tale.

After suffering with a life-long hearing loss Lou was implanted in April and is now using a Cochlear Kanso 2. Like most cochlear implant recipients, he mentions how he waited too long to get a CI. The misconceptions held him back and it was only after a friend received a CI did Lou understand the potential for getting out of the isolation of deafness and into the world of sound.

His dedication to rehabilitation is a factor to his rapid success. For a man who understands dedicated training it should come as no surprise. There is a lot to learn here about that dedication to perfecting his hearing and speech.

Lou is also the first recipient I have interviewed with experience with the Kanso 2. There is insight to this device that candidates who are deciding which Cochlear processor to choose will find helpful.

Lou Ferrigno: My name is Lou Ferrigno, and today is July 26th, 2021. Right now, presently, I'm in Englewood, Colorado.

Richard: Lou, I understand from what I've read, you had a hearing loss from an infection when you were very young. I think one of the things that intrigued me was the fact that you said you were bullied when you had a hearing loss. Could you tell me a little bit about that? I can't imagine somebody bullying you. It must've been an interesting experience.

Lou Ferrigno: Well, at a young age, I used to wear the old-fashioned hearing aid. I went to parochial school. A lot of kids made fun of me, because at the time I had a very severe speech impediment. It was difficult for people to understand when I communicated. I was very skinny as a kid. I wasn't big. I got beat up a lot because I was afraid to defend myself, believe it or not. My father was a police lieutenant. When I go home, I tell my father what happened. He would give me another beating because he said, "Don't come home and you can't fight for yourself." I'd say to myself, "I'm here with this problem, my hearing problem," and children do not have the psychological defenses to defend themselves. I went through that period, went to school and I was always known... People they, "Oh Lou, the deaf kid. That mute, this and that stuff."

Lou Ferrigno: For me, I kept going along because I didn't want to feel sorry for myself. But then eventually I discovered bodybuilding and fitness and that started my journey just changed my whole life because being bullied as a kid, I wanted to work out, be strong because I want to be able to defend myself because I grew up in a tough neighborhood and I got pushed around a lot. I got beat up a lot. Sometimes they would take their finger and flip the hearing aid out of my ear just to be mean because I had the old-fashioned hearing aid. That to me brought so much shame. Sometimes I was too quiet by myself, I would pray to God saying, "I can't keep living like this." Then when I discovered bodybuilding, that gave me the ammunition to be able to build the body, able to change my life.

Richard: Was it a Charles Atlas advertisement in the comic book? What was the thing that flipped you over?

Lou Ferrigno: It's funny, it wasn't Charles Atlas in a comic book. I remember, I looked at it, but I was poor as a kid. I begged my father, "Buy me one of those," he wouldn't. What I did as a kid, I had friends of mine. They had weights, sometimes I would try to lift their weights. I wanted them, to have my own weights. I did, I would go to the junkyard, I would get a pail and I filled it with cement, I put the pole in the middle, so it gets hard. I made myself my own makeshift barbell. For example, I'd get a pail of half full, three quarters, maybe different sizes and made my own barbell there because I couldn't afford it because I was so determined to have my friend had to have weights because then I discovered Muscle Magazine. I'd see the guys like Mr. Universe flexing and I said, "Wow, why can't I be like this?" Because it's a very masculine thing back then.

Richard: You started building your body up. Now, how many years until you won Mr. Universe? How many years of training did you go through?

59

Lou Ferrigno: I started bodybuilding maybe about 12 or 13. I won the Mr. Universe when I was 21, the youngest one to win the IBB Mr. Universe, I've won it twice. I won Teenage American, Mr. America, Mr. International and your favorite governor, Arnold Schwarzenegger.

Richard: Now, all this time, do you have this hearing loss, and you were building up your body, obviously getting bigger and people weren't going to pick on you anymore. My question is basically when you had the hearing loss, you now have won this title twice. You start to build a career. How was your hearing loss affecting that career?

Lou Ferrigno: Well, when I won the Mr. Universe competition, they could not use my interview because my speech was not understandable. Then I realized, I had to do something about my speech. I studied phonetics. I've learned to speak by the hearing of my tone. This way, I didn't want to sound like a deaf person. I wanted to speak the best I can. It was a long, hard journey because I've learned to read lips when I was very young, but the speech therapy, I've gone to speech therapy for many years because it's a lot of sounds we hear, but we say it differently compared to the way it's written.

Lou Ferrigno: I had to endure that. Sometimes, I put marbles in my mouth and try to speak very clearly with marbles in my mouth, to say each word. Because at the time, my speech was like monotone. I sounded like "My name is Lou Ferrigno," but I did not have the inflection like I have now. That made a big difference. In Hollywood, they always put the stigma and limitations. You could play a body role, but you can't play a good acting role because speech was the problem. But I never wanted to feel that I have this deficit. I'm going to do something about it, which I did. That was my journey back then to take me where I am now, especially now with a cochlear implant.

Richard: Your motivation, you're obviously a highly motivated guy. You spent eight or nine years building up for the competition. I read somewhere; you were doing bodybuilding five hours a day which is a huge amount of time. As a motivated person, you now have a cochlear implant. It's been about four months now. We're going to talk about that activation in a second, but I'm very curious, how much time a day do you spend in rehabilitation to get the results you want?

Lou Ferrigno: Almost every day, before I went three times a day, I think are called the Angel App where you have different words and you must distinguish the words, which one is the correct word. To me at the beginning, it was challenging. But then over time got easier and easier because it's just like working out. The good thing about [inaudible 00:06:34] for me to do this because I trained this body to build this body. It's easy for me to have the motivation and the discipline to do that. I was amazed that over the course, how I was hearing better and better, very exciting for me, it's incredible. Now, that's my bad ear. I have 115 decibel loss in the left ear. That took one ear, how well I can hear. Could you imagine when I had the second one?

Richard: Oh my gosh, you're unbelievable. You're an inspiration. By doing this podcast, you're going to inspire more people than you can imagine, because this is not print. My experience is those who listen to these podcasts or read the transcripts, tend to move forward. We get them off the fence. The next topic I wanted to ask, what was the day that you decided to come off the fence and go forward and get a cochlear implant?

Lou Ferrigno: Well, a friend of mine had a similar situation. He had a profound hearing loss. He lost his hearing when he was seven. It got progressively worse. He did a lot of research, and he got a cochlear implant and I saw how well he was going to hear. Now for me, I was at the point that I couldn't improve my hearing anymore with hearing aids. Good hearing aids, you are very limited because it doesn't give you the clarity, like cochlear does so I made the decision. I said, "Why not? Because I'm going to be 70 years old." I said, "I want to wait till I'm to 85, 90." The only thing going to change is your self-taken action to do something about it. I'm very competitive. I just started to get the cochlear and I was determined to hear better, but I'm just amazed that I should've done it sooner.

Lou Ferrigno: I wish I could have done it 10 years ago. But back then people were saying that, "You have a cochlear implant, it doesn't work, you can never go back to a hearing aid. A doctor can't make promises because everyone is different." I was terrified. I was terrified to death before I had the surgery, but I didn't want to tell anybody about it. I was literally terrified. For two times, I was supposed to have the surgery was canceled because of COVID, because of other circumstances. Finally, when I got the chance to do it a third time, I have less fear. I just want to get over with it. It's amazing how, when you hear different sounds, you never hear with a hearing aid like a refrigerator, people whispering. This morning, I hear a fly in my hotel room. I was in the [inaudible 00:08:54] Hotel staying [inaudible 00:08:55]. Yeah. Basically, if I could track that down, I'm doing damn good.

Richard: It's so interesting to me that I waited 35 years, but the misconceptions kept going on and on and on. In fact, I have a YouTube channel and one of the videos I did was for the medical professionals because medical professionals have no clue what cochlear implants are. My short video, five-minute video is dispelling the myths about cochlear implants and hoping that medical professionals will pay attention. It's just amazing. As far as waiting too long, I've gone to seminars for Cochlear. The first question they asked is, "Who regrets having a cochlear?" Nobody raised their hand. The second question is, "Who wishes they had done it sooner," and a hundred hands will go up. It's not an uncommon story. What we're trying to do here is that people know you don't have to wait. My next question is your two sides. One, you had it done. What's left on the other side now? How much [crosstalk 00:10:05] you have left?

Lou Ferrigno: I still have a hearing aid in the right ear.

Richard: You don't need a cochlear implant in that side?

Lou Ferrigno: Eventually, I'd like to, because I feel with two of them, why not have better hearing? This left ear is 115 decibel hearing loss. My right ear is 110. If I can hear this well with 115 decibel hearing loss, I just want to be able to appreciate music more and able to hear better sound because this is just one ear. Most people, they listen out of their right ear. They talk on the phone with the right ear, but I've never really talked on the phone with the left ear, now I can talk [crosstalk 00:10:38].

Richard: Are you listening to music again through the cochlear implant?

Lou Ferrigno: Trying to listen to music, I'm starting to understand the word now by listening very carefully. But I think once I have two of them, it'll make a big difference, the main thing for me is the clarity.

Richard: Yes. The speech clarity is first, and just to tip when you're learning to listen to music that we remember, you go to YouTube and choose a song you remember and use the word with lyrics because the brain kicks in better if it knows the lyrics that you're listening to, do try that.

Lou Ferrigno: That's why it gave me more confidence in my speech. That's more important to me than anything, my own speech. Because right now, as I'm speaking to you, you would never assume I'm hard of hearing. I'm just saying that before I had the cochlear implant, my speech wasn't quite as clear as now. There may be like a five, 10% difference.

Richard: You couldn't hear yourself speaking before? Now you can hear yourself.

Lou Ferrigno: Correct, but before I had to say the words carefully because more memorization, but with the cochlear implant, it will come more naturally.

Richard: Absolutely, it does because now you've had the cochlear implant for four months. Is sound improving every day or do you think you hit a plateau?

Lou Ferrigno: It's improving every day. I think I still have much to learn because especially now, I fly a lot on airplanes and it's amazing that if I take my hearing aid out, I'm going to watch something on the computer subtitled. With the cochlear implant, I can hear what the airplane is doing, or the captain is saying. They talk randomly fast, I could understand what they're saying compared to the hearing aid, because the hearing aid, sometime [inaudible 00:12:15] surrounding the cochlear does more of what you call, differentiate.

Richard: I just went to a charity function last week, which was a happy hour. The room was packed with 200 people. Because of the Smart app from Cochlear I was able to carry on conversations without any problem whatsoever. When you get two of them, you'll do even better.

Lou Ferrigno: When you got the second one, did you see a big advantage?

Richard: I got them both done at the same time. I had nothing to lose. My audiogram looked like a stiff in a morgue. There was nothing there. Like you, when you screwed up my courage to move ahead, the doctor said to me, "Why don't you do two of them? You have nothing to lose." I did it. I was scared.

Lou Ferrigno: I can imagine, but you had no hearing. How long did this go on for before you decided to get the implant?

Richard: 35 years, but I decided to get the implant when I was qualified for, when I moved to Florida. The doctor said, "You're qualified for both." I was so scared. I pushed the operation five months out because I wanted to be sure I wasn't making a rash decision. Therefore, I do what I do to let people know, don't make my mistake. Nothing to fear. If you have nothing to lose and if a doctor is willing to operate on you, you will hear again. The question is how much hearing you will get is never a guarantee. But once the doctors say, "It's okay to operate, you're going to hear." This is the message I constantly work to get out there. Don't be afraid.

Lou Ferrigno: What caught my attention, was that Rush Limbaugh lost his hearing. He went completely deaf I think because he was taking a lot of pain medication. I was amazed that when he had the cochlear implant, he was still able to conduct himself doing radio interviews. I'm saying to myself, "Wow, this is fantastic," because I would assume that he couldn't hear, maybe had difficulty hearing, but that caught my attention.

Richard: That's a very interesting point. Rush discouraged me from getting it for years because he said that he couldn't distinguish male and female voices. It gave me the excuse not to move ahead for many years. I would read his transcript. I couldn't hear him on the radio. I found out later that his first implant was not entirely successful. They could only get maybe 10 or 11 electrodes. He was able to hear, but he couldn't distinguish. The second one may have been more successful. It depends on which day of the week you caught that message. I do have another question for you, you chose Cochlear, why did you choose Cochlear Corporation over any other company?

Lou Ferrigno: I have a friend who did a lot of research and he thought that Cochlear was the best because his sister had it done when and she wasn't hearing that well. Of all the research he's done, that's why it convinced me because I never read much about Cochlear before. I know there were different companies, but then eventually I started to do research, reading that Cochlear is the best and it's best [it has a lot to do with the staff too, because if you have a poor audiologist, It's a team effort here because you're putting your life in somebody's hand. Cochlear to me, has this distinction because what he's been through, because I want to be with the best.

Richard: I must tell you of all the interviews I've done, you're the first person using the Kanso 2, it's a relatively new device. Are you happy with it? What's a pro or con? Is it retaining itself when you're moving around a lot? When you exercise? Tell me a little bit about it?

Lou Ferrigno: the only thing, I just hope in the future they make a little thinner, but right now, not a problem. I can train with it. I do everything, but sometimes I'm getting off the plane, if I must lean forward, if I hid it. What's interesting is that people look at me and they said, "What is that?"

Lou Ferrigno: I tell them what it is, and we have a conversation about it once having a hearing aid then they say, "I'm fine," and just try to hide the situation. Because when I was young, I was telling her that when I was in my 20s, when I go to a discotheque, I wanted a girl more than anything. I was so shy. Sometimes, we would hold each other, she would be kissing me. She would touch me here. I just kept turning my head. She thought maybe I had a twitching habit, or something was wrong with me. She goes, "What's wrong?" I said, "Nothing." I kept turning my head the other way, because I felt that she found out I had a hearing aid, I'll be rejected.

Richard: Lou, I appreciate your time. Do you have anything you would like to tell the listeners about your experience? Anything, message you'd like to give them before we sign off?

Lou Ferrigno: I would say that they'll have no more fear about it because there's a movie that came out about cochlear implant. They made it look like a Frankenstein surgery, which it isn't, because to me it was a minimum two-hour surgery. I had maybe 5% pain and then it's just cutting under the skin. It's not like they must cut your head open. Then once you have this implant in your head, they never have to go back. The only thing that changes is the external processor on the outside.

Richard: It's been a pleasure. I really do appreciate your time. I'm sure, as I said before, "People are going to listen to this and move forward." You've done good work for society. Oh, you know one thing I found very interesting, you were an icon for the deaf community. Has anything changed since you got a cochlear implant? Have they been angry at you? Have you gotten negative feedback?

Lou Ferrigno: No because I do a lot of signing lately. I've done a lot of signing, the people come up, they say, "We've seen you being emotional about the cochlear." They congratulate me. Then people also wearing hearing aid, sometimes they have bad hearing, and they say, "Well, I'm thinking about doing it." I haven't received anything negative. I'll be honest with you; I haven't heard any negative comment. I'm sure they don't want to make a negative comment to me because I'm not a little kid anymore.

Richard: They wouldn't survive five seconds. I got it. It's okay. There's always been a conflict between the deaf community and those who try to leave it by getting a cochlear implant and that conflict is diminishing with time. I was just curious about your own personal experience.

Lou Ferrigno: Don't get me wrong. I met people that need a cochlear implant, they don't want to do it. I try to convince them. They're just happy being deaf. That's their choice. Life is about choice. Do you want to make that choice? Fine.

Richard: I agree with you 100%. Lou, thank you so much for your time.

LOU FERRIGNO PART 2

One of the more frequent questions that candidates for cochlear implants have been about rehabilitation.

Once a candidate receives the implant and is activated by their audiologist, the initial sounds might be robotic or sound like Mickey Mouse. Commitment to doing rehabilitation exercises is key to getting the best results. Your brain needs to learn to hear again and the more one does the rehabilitation programs, sounds will normalize better and faster.

Just over a year ago, I was honored to have the opportunity to talk with Lou Ferrigno about his new cochlear implant and his experiences that let up to his decision to get one.

Recently I heard him participate in a video presentation and I was amazed at the improvement in his diction. In June 2022, I met him at the Hearing Loss Association of America convention in Tampa and again impressed with the improvement.

He graciously agreed to do a follow-up interview with me. The results are best demonstrated by listening to parts one and two for comparison.

He also talks about his decision to seek out his options to move forward to get a cochlear implant for his second side.

Thank you Lou Ferrigno for your insights and congratulations on the improvements.

Rehabilitation never ends. Lou's story is a reminder this hearing journey is not a race but requires dedication to getting the best hearing you can achieve.

Richard:Okay, good morning. Today, we're talking part two interview with Lou Ferrigno, so if you would just start by stating your name, the date, and where you are.

Lou Ferrigno: Yeah. My name is Lou Ferrigno and today is July 13th. I'm living now in the central coast in California.

Richard: I appreciate your time. I wanted to do this interview because it was one year ago. We did part one and you had just received your cochlear implant and you were activated, and your voice was still a little foggy at that time. Recently, I heard you do a video presentation, and then I went to Tampa for the HLAA convention for the question and answers, and your voice has improved so much. I really wanted to concentrate this time on talking about rehabilitation because you are a champion. I have to tell you over the past year, I've referred more people to your interview than anybody else.

Lou Ferrigno: Oh, thank you.

Richard: You've inspired dozens of people to move forward, so I really appreciate your time. Let's talk a little bit about where you are today versus a year ago, in terms of how you feel about what you're doing.

Lou Ferrigno: Well, today, speech, it's much more improved, especially doing all the rehab exercises. It takes five to six months for the cochlear to adapt to almost 100%, and that's why, especially when it comes to the acting and filming and different things, different sounds, everything, I hear everything much clearer, and especially I hear my own voice clearer, meaning that, for example, before you could detect a speech impediment in my voice, but now I think it's very minimal.

But the big change is the fact that I'm getting used to the cochlear, and as a matter of fact, tomorrow, I'm seeing Jordan at House Hearing Clinic. We're talking about getting the second one, to do a hearing test on my right ear, because I'm 70 now, there's a chance I may be losing more of my right hearing. I'm curious to find out tomorrow. But it's been a wonderful life-changing experience, especially now that I'm able to monitor my own voice without thinking about it, without struggling like I used to. That's the big difference.

Richard: I understand that. I struggled for 35 years, totally deaf. I had to regulate the volume of my voice by watching the facial cues of the person I was talking to. You no longer have to do that. What did you do exactly? Can you talk a little bit about rehabilitation, how you got your voice to improve?

Lou Ferrigno: Well, besides the Angel Sounds it had what you call Co-Pilot, for example, that I've learned listening to TED, learning to listen to different conversations, because they give you three questions and you listen to a conversation ... I think five minutes ... and then the different questions, you have to answer each question. For example, they give you direction, or, for example, if you order food, if the conversation is between two or three people, and then later on, you have to answer these questions, that was part of the rehab.

Also, the beginning was tough because I had to learn to differentiate different words, to pick out the right, correct word out of four words. So, for me, it was like 50-60%. It got to a point that was no more than 100%, but now the conversation's much easier because you work up for a single word up to different consonants different sounds at the beginning and the end, that eventually goes to conversation, which is fantastic because when you listen to the conversation, it sounds so different compared to a hearing aid.

Richard: It's an interesting point because people who are considering a cochlear implant, whether it's a single or bilateral, are often afraid of the amount of rehabilitation. But my question is, did you ever get discouraged while you were doing it?

Lou Ferrigno: I would say the very beginning when I first used a different app, I was kind of nervous because my brain was not adapting as quick. It's just like when you to go to school, when you study it gets easier and easier, but you've got to have the right attitude, the positive attitude. But it's a rewarding experience. It's not like you have to do it; it's something that if you do it, it only improves your hearing and it's enjoyment involvement. When you hear better and better, it makes you much more excited. It's not like going to a gym, for example, so you want to train for one year for competition. This is completely different because you're building different steps, you reach to level you want to get to, and for me, it's fun, exciting. Also, you've got to have a positive attitude and the determination to want to do it.

Richard: What about dealing in social situations? Is that much easier for you now or are you still having confusion with sound?

Lou Ferrigno: It's much easier. But the thing is, I do tell people I have a cochlear implant and then it takes the pressure off you because if you're having a conversation with people, for example, for years, I never wanted to tell people I had hearing loss or wore hearing aids because I was afraid of the rejection.

But now it's a conversational piece. When I talk about cochlear implants, they're excited to hear about it, but the most important thing is you're taking pressure off yourselves. That's the most powerful thing, because once you have pressure on yourself, then you could be detrimental to yourself.

Richard: I understand exactly what you're talking about because so many people want to hide that hearing loss because we just started a new Facebook site called Hearing Loss: The Emotional Side, and we've got well over a thousand people within five weeks. People are discussing this kind of thing: "I'm afraid of exposing my hearing loss", "I'm afraid to do this or that," and they're pouring their emotions out on the page. Do you have an emotional change since you received cochlear implants that you can describe?

Lou Ferrigno: Well, especially at home now, especially when I talk to my family, I can listen to them when I'm walking away behind my back, whereas I had to constantly lean forward and to constantly use more effort to listen to conversation, especially when hearing the children, home, the kids screaming and the wife and everything. It's much easier because it's almost like, for example, we live in my childhood and I'm able to hear the thing that I wish I heard when I was a child.

Richard: That's absolutely fabulous. Now, I noticed at the question and answer at Tampa you did, you were using your phone on your right side. Is that your hearing aid side?

Lou Ferrigno: I go back and forth because I can use both the hearing aid and the cochlear on the phone. The reason why I use it on the phone is because sometimes if they call me, it's easier to listen to the phone if I go to the cochlear. Then I have to click the mute button. But my goal to get the second implant eventually and I could have two which makes it much easier. I hear much easier with the cochlear compared to the hearing aid. Big difference. I mostly use the cochlear, but then sometimes I switch because depending on if I want to listen to something on the computer or a specific thing, I switch it around.

Richard:

Okay. Now you're considering going to bilateral. I'd like to talk about that a little bit: your hesitations, what's changed over the past year, and why you're looking into it.

Lou Ferrigno: Well, the thing is that when you have a cochlear implant and you have a hearing aid at the same time, it's not a very good marriage because sometimes they take away from the cochlear. Then when you want to go with the cochlear and then you say to yourself, "Wow. I hear so much better than hear ..." If I had it my way, I wish I could just have the cochlear, take the hearing aid out, and I could manage. I could get around about the same, but I'd rather maximize what I have right now.

I talked to some people after I saw you the next day at the airport, and I met a woman that eventually she went bilateral, and she said before she had the same situation, like you and I, and she told me when she got the second one, she was able to hear. In other words, it gave more depth to 360 degrees instead of just one ear. I'm sure you're familiar with that.

Richard: When you did rehabilitation, did you take the hearing aid out while you were listening all day? Or did you do it for a few hours a day? Do you remember?

Lou Ferrigno: In the beginning, I would say maybe half a day because they told me only do only a couple hours and take a break, but it got to a point that I would continue to do the rehabilitation. It wasn't that tiresome because at the beginning your brain gets tired after lifting so much; you need to give yourself a break. Now, it's not a problem for me anymore. But sometimes I take the hearing aid out, and I just listen with the cochlear.

Richard: That's good because actually this morning, I was referred to a woman who was about to get the first one, she has a hearing aid on the other side, and she was asking me about rehabilitation. I'm sure she's going to want to listen to this or read this interview. Do you have anything else you'd like to add to the people? I know you've done a tremendous job. You've been so unbelievably inspiring. How does it feel to know that people move forward because of your intervention?

Lou Ferrigno: I feel great because these people are just saying that I wish I had done it 10 years sooner because in fact why suffer? Because I'm not 21; I'm not 19 years old. But the most important thing is that it makes up what you didn't have before. It's almost like people go back to school.

They never got an education. They go back to school, get an education. You're able to go back. That's why a lot of people, sometimes they have one cochlear ... I have a friend of mine who has a cochlear. He doesn't want to get the second one; he's happy with one. Some people are happy with one, but my situation I want to maximize, I want to have a 100%.

Richard: Congratulations. I think it's going to be fabulous. Once you have stereo hearing, you're going to wonder why you waited a year. Now, most people do wait six months to one year, so you're right within that framework. I had them both done at the same time, so I can't tell about my experience that way. That was easier because I could rehabilitate two ears at the same time.

Lou Ferrigno: Yeah. How was your speech before you had the bilateral.

Richard: Well, people thought I was Russian because of my accent. But I'll tell you what was very interesting is that I moved here seven years ago, and I left a lot of my friends in New York. After I got my cochlear implant, I would be talking to them on the phone and they would say, "Richard, your voice sounds so much better." It does, in my experience, it makes a big difference. And as I've said, listening to you a year ago and people are going to be reading or listening to both these interviews to make a comparison, and you are light years ahead of where you were a year ago.

Lou Ferrigno: That's why tomorrow I'll go to the ear clinic to do the testing for the second one because after one year you have to go for the testing. They basically said, "You're definitely a candidate for the second one." So, I'd be curious to find out, because my right ear, I am losing my natural hearing. That's why tomorrow I want to see, because I want to get to a point that was explained that when come to your natural hearing, when you get older, sometimes you could have a drop. One morning, you could wake up, you could lose like 15-20%. It can happen. I want to be ahead of the game.

Richard: It's true, because losing any degree of natural hearing is so frightening to people. I tell the story of a woman I mentored in Mississippi, 3% in one ear, zero in the other, and the surgeon wanted to operate on her so-called good ear, and she took one year to decide. Losing natural hearing is something people really want to hold onto. It's a big step for them to understand your story and I appreciate that.

Lou Ferrigno: But I think it's a good point you brought up because people that, for example, start to lose some of their hearing, I think in older, even different age, they should consider cochlear. Don't wait. Don't procrastinate because then it'd be more detrimental.

Richard: Lou, thank you so much for your time.

Lou Ferrigno: You're welcome.

CHAPTER 6 MARY BETH NAPOLI

A TEACHER OF THE DEAF GETS A LESSON FROM HER STUDENTS

Why would a teacher of the deaf, with her own severe hearing loss, wait years to get her own cochlear implant? I asked Mary Beth Napoli, a bilateral Med-El cochlear implant recipient and a member of the Facebook group, Bilateral CI Warrior, to share her unique perspective.

She struggled with her own severe hearing loss for decades. She had years of working with cochlear implant recipients who needed auditory training after implantation.

She witnessed the remarkable results her student experienced but as many cochlear implant candidates who have walked the path towards getting hearing help, she was fearful of losing her miniscule amount of residual hearing.

She discusses the reasons why she chose MED-EL from her point of view and the surgeon's.

Although Mary Beth's unique medical history is complex her story is invaluable to candidates who are considering and researching cochlear implants. Her results are remarkable. She enjoys music and to be able to fully participate in all activities with hearing. She loves that she is no longer dependent on others to interpret the conversations around her.

Mary Beth Napoli: My name is Mary Beth Napoli. Today is June 9th, 2021. And I am in the northeast corner of New York State, Plattsburgh, New York.

Richard: Mary Beth, tell me a little bit about your hearing loss, the history of it. Did they know what caused it? I'm giving you the floor right now.

Mary Beth Napoli: I was born with typical hearing and when I was 13, I failed a hearing screening at school and that started the tracking of my hearing loss. Otosclerosis runs in my dad's family, and it turns out that I have otosclerosis. It just began earlier than normal in me and progressed faster than what is typical. My hearing loss got worse and progressed starting at age 13. Every year, when I would go back for a hearing test, it would have dropped, and they were really just monitoring it. No one ever talked to me about an option for hearing aids, even with a moderate conductive hearing loss back then. Hearing aids were never discussed, and I definitely had the opinion that the plan was to monitor my hearing until it got to a point where a stapedectomy surgery could be a viable option.

Mary Beth Napoli: By the time I was in high school though, my hearing loss was interfering with my day-to-day life, and I had one ear that was better than the other, so I would always do the hallway dance and make sure that my friends were on my better side, so I had a better chance of hearing them. When I went to undergrad, my hearing loss was the big issue because the classes were in lecture halls. One professor way down at the bottom and then stadiums seating with all of us, and I couldn't hear the professor. The professor kept turning around, so I couldn't speech read the professor. I didn't have hearing aids. Whenever she wrote in her notebook, I copied in mine and whatever the professor wrote on the board, I copied down. And I read and read and read before I showed up to class to try to have a better chance of following everything.

Mary Beth Napoli: It was during undergrad, I think it was between my junior and senior year in undergrad that, finally, we were going to do a stapedectomy on my worst year. I had the surgery, and it was a success for one month. And then I developed a fistula and then they had to go in and patch that hole and redo the stapedectomy. And that was a success for three months. And then I developed another fistula and by then, a different surgeon went in and put a very strong graft into patch, so no more holes would develop and did not insert a prosthesis. And that is when my life with hearing aids began.

Richard: What kind of hearing aids did you get at the time?

Mary Beth Napoli: In my 20s, I don't remember the brand name of the first hearing aids I had.

Richard: Were they behind the ear-

Mary Beth Napoli: ... I just remember hating them.

Mary Beth Napoli: Behind the ear.

Mary Beth Napoli: Behind-the-ear hearing aids. I wore behind-the-ear hearing aids almost exclusively. At one time, I did a canal hearing aid for a short period of time. Years later, I developed many ear symptoms in the ear that had had all these surgeries and complications. And in order to get rid of all the vertigo issues and me stable in my life, like to walk around without getting sick and be able to do normal things, we did a transcanal labyrinthectomy in that ear. And I knew I would lose all the hearing in that ear with that surgery, and I did lose all the hearing in that ear, but it also got rid of all of the symptoms that I was having with many years, so it was a great blessing.

Mary Beth Napoli: At that time, I started to use a BiCROS hearing aid that would send sound from my ear that couldn't hear anything to the ear that needed amplification with a hearing aid. And that was a WIDEX BiCROS hearing aid, analog hearing aid. And I used that for years until hearing aids advanced to digital hearing aids. And then, the option to cross the sound was more like wearing a Phonak receiver attached to a digital hearing aid and a Phonak transmitter that resembled a hearing aid on the ear that couldn't hear. And I really did not like that set up at all.

Richard: But why?

Mary Beth Napoli: The digital hearing aid that I had bought at that time, which I think may still have been WIDEX, had such great sound quality, but the sound that was crossing over was so inferior.

Mary Beth Napoli: It was like, I spent a lot of money for this really expensive hearing aid, and then I was downgrading it by having it also merged with this CROS sound quality. I stopped wearing the CROS, and I just wore the hearing aid and then had one ear, one side that could hear nothing and had nothing picking up sound from that side, and then the other ear that still was advancing with otosclerosis and had never been operated on. I kept needing more and more powerful hearing aids on my one ear as time went by. And eventually, we got to the point where no hearing aid. We tried all of the brands. We just tried every option there was. None of the hearing aids could help me because my dynamic range was so small. It was 15 decibels. By the time, the sound was loud enough that I could hear it, a tiny bit louder than that was painful.

Mary Beth Napoli: I was constantly saying to people, "You need to speak louder to me so I can hear you." And then I was saying, "That's too loud." It was really frustrating mess. Eventually, I was limited to really communicating one-on-one. Using the auditory input from the hearing aid and speech reading a person at the same time, and I'm a teacher at that time. I was working as a teacher of the deaf, and I was working with kids who were in mainstream programs. And almost all of the kids were kids who listened and spoke in classes where everyone spoke. The listening demands at work were just overwhelming. By the time I came home from work, I was exhausted. I would turn off my hearing aid and just read a book in complete silence. I didn't want any more auditory input at all. I was so frustrated.

Richard: My question is, were you isolating yourself from people at that time or did you have friends who would understand that you had a situation? Were people very understanding about it?

Mary Beth Napoli: I really am very lucky. My spouse is a child of deaf adults and is fluent in sign language, and I am fluent in sign language. At home communication was never a problem because at home we could just sign. Our friends were understanding. Only a couple of our friends actually sign. Most of our friends do not know any sign at all, and so they were understanding and supportive. But no matter how understanding and supportive they were, it's really lonely to be in a group of people that you love and be unable to feel connected and participate in what is going on around you. I appreciate everything our friends and family did to help me and try to keep me up.

Richard: When did you decide to go for a cochlear implant then? How many years did it take until you decided to get that?

Mary Beth Napoli: It took getting to that level of isolation and desperation. And to be perfectly honest, as a teacher of the deaf, I was working with students with cochlear implants for years, and I was providing their aural rehab and I was seeing the success that they were having, but I was hesitant to pursue a cochlear implant for myself. And this is why it's those cochlear implants simulations that are available online. You go when you listen to what speech sounds like with a cochlear implant. This is what music sounds like with a cochlear implant. I didn't want that. It sounds terrible.

Richard: I have stopped YouTube from several incidents when they played those pseudoscientific clips about music and speech with a cochlear implant. I've complained and I've said to them, "It's going to discourage people from getting a cochlear implant with pseudoscience." What you're saying absolutely hits home.

Mary Beth Napoli: There was an event that we were attending that made me decide it was time to pursue a cochlear implant. We were at a close friend's wedding, and it was a beautiful ceremony. I was having a very difficult time speech reading everyone at the event. There was music and a dance floor, and I could not even figure out the beat of the music. I couldn't dance because I had no idea where the beat even was. In that moment, I decided I had to do something. And so right after that, I called and made my appointment with a CI surgeon to see if a cochlear implant was a possibility for me, and it took all that time. I'd like to say, if I had to do it all over again, I would have gotten a cochlear implant sooner because they're just amazing and life changing. But the reality is, I probably would have waited just as long to be mentally and emotionally ready to embrace the cochlear implant journey and be willing to put in the aural rehab time.

Richard: It took me 35 years. How long did it take you to make the decision?

Mary Beth Napoli: Well, it's a slippery slope. When did my one hearing aid get to the point where I was no longer functioning well? A long time. We would be at a large family event for holiday. And then at night, I would say to my spouse, "Okay, catch me up. What's going on in everybody's life?" And she'd fill me in on absolutely everything that I missed, which was absolutely everything that happened. So, it took me a long time to get there. Exactly how long? I don't know. I'd say I probably should have pursued the cochlear implant 10 years before I did, but it took a long time for me to be ready.

Richard: When I received my cochlear implants, I became a volunteer because I wanted to play my experience forward. And I would go to these training seminars, and the leader of the seminar would say, "Who regrets getting a cochlear implant?" And nobody would raise a hand. Then he would say, "Who wishes they had done it sooner?" And 50 people would be waving their arms. It's true. What's water under the bridge is water under the bridge. We understand that you can't go back, but by having these conversations, I'm hoping people who are hearing this for the first time, hear our stories, and stop sitting on the fence, and get off and move off the fence.

Mary Beth Napoli: It's difficult because when you talk with people who are thinking about getting cochlear implants, there's a level of hearing that most of them have that they don't want to lose. They don't want to lose something. In fact, cochlear implants were complete win for me, not some magical win that you see on YouTube. I was not one of those people who heard speech at activation. I did a lot of aural rehab, but I have never heard this well since I was a young teenager decades and decades ago. I am enjoying the absolute best hearing, best music, best speech, and noise that I've heard in many decades. It's just life-changing.

Richard: I'd like to take you back to a point you've decided to move forward. And I assume you had the same, maybe not, scenario that most of us do in regard to the audiologist. Then she dumps a bunch of brochures on your lap and says, "Choose one. Choose a company." And I call that the document dump. I'd like to know your experience. What are you wearing and how did you choose it?

Mary Beth Napoli: I went to a large cochlear implant center in New York City. I wanted a CI surgeon who was not going to be taken back by the surgeries that I had already had in my right ear. I had heard so many times from doctors that they had never seen this before. I thought by going to a very large CI center, I had a better chance that the surgeons will have been familiar with something similar to this or be ready to embrace it and find a way forward. When I did, the surgeon was interested in putting a cochlear implant in my longstanding deaf ear, the ear that heard nothing for 24 years. So I went through the imaging that you do beforehand and went through the two-hour audiological assessment that qualifies you and all of that. What ended up happening is they do give you the binders for the three FDA-approved brands of cochlear implants in the US and tell you to look at it and it's your choice, and then you come back.

Mary Beth Napoli: Now, my appointments may have been different than most people because my cochlear implant center is five hours away from my home, so they were very kind to me, and they scheduled things on the same day when they could. I was going to be seeing the surgeon and doing the brand selection all on the same day. And when I saw this surgeon, it wasn't great news. He wasn't sure whether or not they would be able to get an electrode array into that cochlea. It was very ossified from otosclerosis, and the imaging did not look good. The way it looked combined with the fact that it had not heard anything at all for 24 years, the prognosis of success with a cochlear implant was really small, and he would not implant me if I would not be satisfied with that ear helping me speech read. The thought was, I would have no open-set speech understanding in that ear, no ability to understand speech if I didn't know the choices of words that were coming.

Mary Beth Napoli: I almost turned it down and it was a very difficult appointment, and I kept going back and forth with whether I should try it or not try it. I'm so thankful for his patience and the time he spent with us that day trying to decide. In the end, I decided what did I have to lose? The ear heard nothing at all. My balance system was already disconnected on that side. So as long as I was willing to take the risk, the usual risks of anesthesia, what did I have to lose? I decided to go forward.

Richard: Was this at NYU? Did you go to NYU?

Mary Beth Napoli: No. I go to New York Eye and Ear of Mount Sinai.

Richard: Okay. Who was the surgeon?

Mary Beth Napoli: That surgeon was Dr. Alexiades at that time.

Mary Beth Napoli: I had two different surgeons on my right and my left because he moved on to become the director at a different CI program after my first surgery. We decided to go forward and then the decision had to be which brand were we going to go forward with? And I actually had that discussion with my surgeon first, instead of my audiologist. I was concerned now that we might not be able to get an electrode array into my cochlea. My discussion focused a hundred percent on which electrode array do you think you have the best chance of getting into my complicated cochlea and in that discussion, that's what led me to MED-EL because my surgeon felt he wanted three electrodes arrays available to him for my surgery. He was going to use a test electrode array that would determine which electrode would really be best.

Mary Beth Napoli: His hope was that the medium electrode array, which is stiff, would work and penetrate through my blockages. If the medium electrode array didn't work, he wanted to use a compressed electrode array, which is just a shorter electrode array that has all the same number of contacts on it. And if that didn't work, he wanted to use a split electrode array where they just drilled two straight lines through your cochlea and put in two straight leads that have the contacts on it. And so MED-EL had the best assortment of electrode arrays that were going to work with my complicated cochlea, so that was the decision right then.

COCHLEARIMPLANTBASICS.COM

Richard: This is a very interesting discussion because when people are trying to choose, it's really not up to the surgeons to determine, it's up to the recipient, except in a case like yours, whether your surgeon feels there's a better chance of success with a particular brand one over the other. You want to describe a little bit about activation day and your life now with cochlear implants. Are you an active person? What kind of results do you get? Mention about you enjoy music again, which is something a lot of recipients are worried about.

Mary Beth Napoli: Right. That's true. I chose MED-EL because of the electrode arrays and at activation, the surgeon was able to get the medium electrode array in, so I was so excited. And then, my hope for activation was that this ear that had heard nothing at all for 24 years would hear beeps from all 12 electrodes. And I was hoping the beeps wouldn't all sound exactly the same because I knew that if they sounded different, I had a better chance of aural rehab. And that's exactly what happened. I heard all 12 of the different beeps, and they did not sound the same. I was a happy camper. After that, the audiologist that I worked with was an awesome audiologist. She turned on the processor for speech, and she started to speak to me. And it just sounded like static and beeps. That's all. Just static and beeps. And then, I was speech reading her and listening to the static and beeps.

Mary Beth Napoli: I noticed that the static and beeps were starting to line up with her syllables, so I was amazed that if she said something that had four syllables, I heard four bursts of static and beeps. I was very, very excited to be hearing in that ear. Since we live five hours away and I'm a teacher of the deaf, so I'm familiar with aural rehab, my spouse and I started training on the way home. I gave three words that were different in number of syllables, like red, yellow, magenta. And then she would say one of those three words and based on whether it was like one burst of static or two or three, I would say the word. And she would tap me once. If I was right. And twice if I was wrong, we used all different things. Fruit, family member names.

Mary Beth Napoli: At one point in the drive, we were working on fruit, and she said something, and I heard yellow. And I was like, "Did you say yellow?" And she's like, "I did say yellow." I'm like, "Were you trying to trick me?" She's like, "I was trying to trick you." And so yellow was the first word I heard. And then I looked away from Jill and then I heard, "Wow." I'm like, "Did you say wow?" She's like, "I did." Then she said, "Far out." I was like, "Did you say far out?" So yellow, wow, and far out were my first open-set speech. It just got better and better. It got better and better every day. I trained a lot. I spent a couple of hours every day in short sessions, training my new ear to hear, and I would wake up in the morning.

Mary Beth Napoli: I couldn't wait to put on my CI and find out what wow moments I had. Our first short phone call whispering in that ear. I mean, it was just amazing. My ear that had not heard anything for 24 years and had a very complicated-looking cochlea ended up being absolutely wonderful cochlear implant ear. Several months out, I could have conversations from two different floors with that ear. I was using the telephone with unknown people. I was recognizing everybody's voice. I could tell if somebody had a cold based on how their voice sounded. And at about the three- or four-month mark, music started to make advances. In the beginning, music was quite a mess. And two notes played on a keyboard sounded exactly the same to me. It was like, "Okay, I'm not ready for that yet."

Mary Beth Napoli: I would listen to music and just pay attention to the part I could get. Like I'm hearing the drums, I'm hearing percussion. I am hearing the bass instruments. I know someone is singing. And it was just like layers that kept peeling away until, finally, I was understanding and enjoying music well. And then I really was feeling like we had benched my best player. My ear that had always heard, had never been operated on, that could not understand hardly anything with the hearing aid, it still had a hearing aid. So as cochlear implant journey advanced, things changed in my brain with paying attention to the hearing aid or the cochlear implant input, and I described it as a dance. At first, the cochlear implant's side was just happy to follow along, and my acoustic gear was the leader. And then, there was this point in time when the two sides were physically fighting with each other in my head, it was so tiring. And then my cochlear implant got so much better. It took the lead, and my hearing aid became like a permanent noisemaker-

Mary Beth Napoli:

... and then I stopped wearing it.

Richard: It's very common. How long did it take before you decide to go for the second side?

Mary Beth Napoli: I was ready for the second side three months after the first side was activated. In my mind, I knew this hearing is so good I want it on both sides of my head, but it was at my six-month appointment after activation that we discussed implanting my second side. And then by the time my second side was scheduled for surgery, there was eight months between the two.

Richard: It's about average. Less than one year is about the average.

Richard: I would like to close out this interview by asking you, do you have any advice for people who are listening, who are researching about cochlear implants now because your viewpoint is very, very important to these people.

Mary Beth Napoli:

My advice to anyone who is considering getting a cochlear implant is to get one. Just do it and reach out, talk to people, listen to people's stories who have all three brands of cochlear implants, and then decide which one you think is going to be best for you.

Richard: I think it's an absolutely excellent interview. Thank you so much for your time.

Chapter 7 Debbie Entsminger

Hearing Problem? I didn't Have a Hearing Problem. Until I Couldn't Deny it Anymore.

Debbie Entsminger's hearing loss was gradual, so she does not know when it began but it was diagnosed when she was in college.

At the time it was a 10% loss. An annoying inconvenience. Next time she was tested it was 20%. With each successive test, her hearing loss grew and grew until it was 80% or more.

Now it was a severe handicap. Debbie persevered and continued her career albeit at a difficult and exhausting pace.

Eventually she considered getting a cochlear implant, but she had a major complication, a condition known as Bing Siebenmann Dysplasia which lessened her chance of a successful activation.

Again, with her deep faith, she moved forward to achieve remarkable results and later decided for a second surgery to become bilateral. She now has 95% speech comprehension.

Richard: Tell me a little bit about your hearing loss. Did you have health issues? What do you think caused your hearing loss?

Debbie Entsminger: Well, I honestly didn't know for the longest time what caused my hearing loss. I didn't even know I had hearing loss to be honest, and I'm not sure exactly when it started. When I was in college, I took an introduction to communications disorders class, they said for extra credit, have the grad students check your hearing. Always one for extra credit, I was like, "Okay." I went and had the hearing test, and while they were doing it, they realized I'd had a 10% loss. And that was the first time I ever knew anything about me having a hearing loss.

Debbie Enstminger: I always knew I liked to sit in the front row, and it would bother me if they put you alphabetically, you had to sit back farther, but I didn't really know why. But a 10% loss was not that much. There were some sounds I couldn't hear, maybe some alarms or things, but I just didn't think it was a big deal. They recommended that I come back again to get it periodically checked. My senior year I went back, and they discovered another 10% had gone. By that point it was a 20% loss, and that's when it began to really impact my life.

Richard: What did you do with that? Or did you look for hearing aids?

Debbie Enstminger: Well, it was interesting. When I met with the otolaryngologist, he sat me down, and he was a friend of the family. At that point I had wanted to go overseas and be a missionary, and he just sat me down and he said, "Deb, you are never going to be fluent in another language. In fact, as you get older, you're going to have a hard time with English." And I was like, "What?" So, that was the first clue I had, this is going to impact my life.

Debbie Enstminger: He made the comment at the time, he said, "Deb, God hasn't done a miracle giving you your hearing back, but he has done one in enabling you to understand by reading lips." And I didn't even know I was lipreading. Then I realized, "Oh, so this is one of the reasons..." I knew it bothered me if people put their hands in front of their mouths when they would talk, but I really was kind of clueless.

Richard: Of course. Okay. You're in college, so you must have been about 22-

Debbie Enstminger: Yes.

Richard: ... when you started realizing it. At what point did you really have to go for hearing aid? Was it 10 years later? How long, do you remember?

Debbie Enstminger: Well, do you know? I didn't go back to graduate school until I was 27. So that would have been five years later. And about halfway through, one of my mom's friends, she said, "Deb, do you think that getting hearing aids might help?" Because by that point it seemed like every four years, I was losing another 10%. By that point I had lost 30% of my hearing, was starting to really notice as a disability. So, she said, "I'll buy you hearing aids."

Richard: Did you get them?

Debbie Enstminger: I got hearing aids, and of course, this is back in 1992, so hearing aids were very different back then, I'd put them on, and I'd go to class, and I would hear the air conditioner, and it would just drown out the sound of the professor's voice. At that point, hearing aids were more of a hindrance than a help. And I tried for probably about a semester, really tried to make them work, but they just were not helping me. And I found I'd do better just to continue with my regular plans of sitting up front so I could keep reading the professor's lips. I never wore hearing aids after that point.

Richard: Okay. Now, you left college, you left graduate school-
Debbie Enstminger: Yes.

Richard: What point did you get hearing aids?

Debbie Enstminger: Believe it or not, I never got hearing aids after that point. I'd just function, continuing to adapt, with lipreading, and just pressed on all the way up until the point where I lost everything. I was still lipreading.

Richard: Well, then, describe your jobs. You had no hearing. You went to work for... It's kind of a little bit of a handicap.

Debbie Enstminger: Well [crosstalk 00:06:32] opened a door for me. I started working with college students in 2000. My husband and I went on staff with a Christian organization working in a campus ministry. My job was meeting with students, just helping them to get to know the Lord and answering their questions about the big issues in life. A lot of what I did was one-on-one.

Debbie Enstminger: But it was really fascinating because I remember one point, just being so frustrated. By this point I had lost 80% of my hearing.

Richard: Oh my God.

Debbie Enstminger: And we had just moved to the University of Florida. There hadn't been a ministry there for eight years. There wasn't anybody waiting in line. No students to meet with us. I would always initiate with people, never knowing if I'd be able to understand them or not. That was a challenge. And it was interesting. I met this one girl and she said, "Oh, would you come lead a Bible study in my scholarship house? Because I would just love to see something take place there, I think it would just pull us all together." And I was like, "Okay, well, see who's interested."

Debbie Enstminger: She gives me a list of 10 girls, and I was so scared, because of course, you know, scholarship houses, it's terrible acoustics. There's nothing on the walls. And I remember showing up, driving up at this scholarship house that first day, and inside I was just like, "Oh, Lord, the only reason I'm going in there is because I believe you exist, but I have no idea how I'm going to do this. I am scared stiff." And I walked in, and the girls are all sitting around this table. And I sat down, and I told them, I said, "Okay. I have no idea how this is going to work, because I have lost 80% of my hearing, and I don't even know how I'm going to understand you."

Debbie Enstminger: The student sitting right next to me was studying speech pathology and ideology and she said, "I'll tell you how it's going to work." And she put her arm around me and looked at the girls, and said, "Not one of you is to open your mouth without raising your hand to capture Deb's attention, because Deb needs to know which lips to look at." And she proceeded to not only teach them how to make it work but to teach me how to make it work. I still use a lot of the skills that she taught me that day in that study, and it was so neat, because that was one of the most special studies, I think, I've ever had.

Debbie Enstminger: It was funny because a lot of the girls, at first, weren't even sure if they wanted to be there. It was so neat because afterwards I felt like the Lord said to me, "Deb, do you know, if you'd gone in there confident, able to hear, "Okay, I'm here to help you guys understand the Bible," they might never have come back. But because you went in weakness, it drew them all in and they were determined to make this work." And it was the neatest thing seeing lives change because of my weakness.

Richard: But did you ever feel that you could no longer continue with your job because of your hearing? Or did you always have the confidence?

Debbie Enstminger: It's interesting. There is this verse in second Corinthians, 9:8, that says, "And God is able to make all grace abound to you, so in all things at all times, having all you need, you will abound in every good work he has for you to do." And I just clung to that, and I just kept crying out, "God, give me the grace. Would you help me figure out a way." Sometimes, towards the end, I would take with me... It's one of these kid things. I can't even remember what it's called. But you can write on it and then erase it.

Debbie Enstminger: And I couldn't even understand a word-

Debbie Enstminger: You just got creative; you know? In learning. And people just saw it as a challenge, I guess.

Richard: It's true that people I interview, one of the things that I like to find out about is their adaptation techniques.

Debbie Enstminger: Yes.

Richard: You found your adaptation technique. I did too. I mean, we're in business, we must do this.

Debbie Enstminger: Yes.

Richard: You never thought about the fact you couldn't do the job anymore. You just found your adaptation techniques.

Debbie Enstminger: Yeah. I just had the strong sense that this was what God wanted me to do, and I may have to get creative. And do you know, it was so amazing, because at first, I was really frustrated. Initially, right out of college, I was ready to go be a pioneer missionary, do whatever God wanted me to do, and so hearing it close that door, but then was a little bit later in life, it was about 14 years later that we went on staff with this ministry. And I was like, "God, you closed the door when I'd only lost 20% of my hearing. Now you wait till I've lost 80% and you have us go on campus doing this. What are you thinking?"

Debbie Enstminger: And there was this guy who came in to speak at the University of Florida, and he had a doctorate in audiology, and he had a doctorate in psychology. He said as people become deaf their world tends to get smaller because of fear and pride. They're afraid of saying the wrong thing, and there's pride. They don't want to ask for help. And as I sat there in that workshop, I just so sensed God was saying to me, "Deb, do you realize? I have you doing this because I love you. I do not want your world to get smaller, so I've put you in a place where you've just got to press into the heart, and you've got to keep trusting me and keep being creative, trying to adapt, and figure this out. And you are just in the process. You are just annihilating fear and pride. Leaning into the challenge." And my world kept getting bigger.

Richard: I can understand that. There must have been something that moved you forward, finally, toward getting a cochlear implant.

Debbie Enstminger: Yes.

Richard: And that's something I'd be very interested in hearing more about.

Debbie Enstminger: It is interesting, because for me the hardest part of hearing loss wasn't not being able to hear as much as it was the brain fatigue. Because lipreading, they say, takes about seven times more effort on your brain's part to process what you're doing. It was probably right around 2012, so about seven years ago, that I really started experiencing the consequences of brain fatigue. That was right about the time when I was losing almost all residual hearing, and I just started realizing I was getting exhausted. My capacity was decreasing and my ability to interact with people, even if I'd press through for one day and spend the day meeting with student after student, the next day you could barely scrape me off the floor.

Debbie Enstminger: I was just like, "Oh my gosh," this is something that I was just really, really struggling with. And I always expected that I was going to end my days completely deaf, do you know? Because I really thought, "That's the way it's going to be," and I had just kind of embraced it, accepted that, and I thought, "Well, you know, either God's going to have me start a ministry with people who are deaf and I'll just interact with them, or maybe he's going to have me start writing." And I'd be okay with that.

Debbie Enstminger: But every time I tried to move in either of those directions, God kept closing the door, and instead leading me to work that involved even more hearing as he had me get trained as a coach. First with coaching people through their strength finder assessment results, through another assessment, EMCOR, then when he led me to get trained as a Paterson LifePlan facilitator, which takes 16 hours in two days with one person, and it's like, "I'm deaf. I don't have this capacity." And you know, I just feel like your life is like a story and God is this master author. And as I zoomed out looking at the story, I was like, "The way God's leading me is not into this quiet direction. It's a direction where there's more hearing. I've got to figure out what can I do?" It's like, "How do you adapt?"

Debbie Enstminger: That was when I had heard about cochlear implant, and that was about the time when I thought, "I wonder if God might want me to pursue these cochlear implants?"

Richard: Do you remember hearing about cochlear implants? Where you first heard about them and how you felt about them when you heard about them?

Debbie Enstminger: Here's the deal. When I first had heard about them, oh, goodness, easy 10-plus years prior to getting them, what happened was is they told me, with my hearing loss, and because it had been so long, they said, "We can't guarantee that you'll regain voice recognition, and you may lose your residual hearing, and we don't know that you'll regain this." This was back probably around 2005, 2007 or something, back in through there.

Debbie Enstminger: I since learned there's also misinformation out there, and you don't always know you're hearing exactly the facts. When I'm thinking about that, I was like, I still had some residual hearing, and I really relied on that. It's kind of like somebody saying, "Well, if you have this surgery, you might lose this residual hearing," and I'm like, "Well, that will plunge me into total deafness quicker, and hearing dogs and birds isn't really going to help me with my job."

Debbie Enstminger: So, I just didn't really consider it. Then when I went... I guess it was around 2014 they told me, "Oh, they've got a new technique that could help conserve, possibly, your residual hearing." They said, "But it's kind of new, so you might want to let the surgeons practice on someone else first." So that was why I was like, "All right, I'll wait a couple years." When I reached this point, it would have been back in summer of 2017, it was time for me to get another exam, just to go and get it checked out. I thought, "Well, all right, I'll go have them check everything out and I'll just ask about cochlear implant."

Debbie Enstminger: By that point, I had absolutely zero hearing that you could measure medically as far as that. It is really an interesting process, because then you've got to go through the process of them doing tests to determine are you a candidate for this? And just waiting to find out. And it was interesting throughout the process, I really wasn't sure. I was like, "Lord, is this something that you really want me to do?" And I just sensed him leading me. "This is a tool, and it's a tool that will help you to be able to continue to engage and do the things that I'm leading you to do."

Debbie Enstminger: I felt like he was having me move forward, and brain fatigue was holding me back. I was like, "If this helps this could be huge."

Richard: But you basically were waiting until all the residual hearing was gone and then you moved forward at that point, because you had almost nothing left at that time.

Debbie Enstminger: That's right. When I went into the doctor, I was like, "So, this is the main thing I want to know. Will cochlear implants help

COCHLEARIMPLANTBASICS.COM

me?" And he looked at me and goes, "Of course they'll help you hear. You're hearing nothing now." And he says, "At least you'll be able to hear dogs bark, birds sing, and all of that. What we don't know is whether you'll regain voice recognition or not." Richard: And did you?

Debbie Enstminger: Oh, my goodness, it has been the most amazing thing. Right now, my last hearing test... I told you before cochlear implants it was zero, my last hearing test, 95% regain of voice recognition- Debbie Enstminger: ... in the sound booth.

Richard: Wow!

Debbie Enstminger: Oh, it has been the most amazing, life-changing experience. I feel like this year has been a year of wonder. Of hearing things, I didn't even know made noises.

Richard: Talk to me about the day of surgery. You were nervous about surgery going into it? Or how did you feel about the surgery itself?

Debbie Enstminger: It made such a difference, having a surgeon that I felt so confident in. And I mean, I just felt so incredibly blessed that I had Dr. Loren Bartels doing my surgery and had talked to other people who told me that he was just topnotch. But also, when I went in for my first visit with Dr. Bartels, I had told my husband before, I said, "You know what drives me crazy? As I go in for audiology visits, otolaryngologist visits, and they put you in a chair that is cemented to the floor and then they sit along the side of the wall, and I just want to keep scooting the chair closer so I can read their lips better."

Debbie Enstminger: With Dr. Bartels, he was amazing, the way his whole setup, he knew how to work with deaf people. He had a screen, and when he would speak into a microphone, and it would transcribe everything he was saying so that you could really understand what he was saying. And he gave you a printed copy of the notes when you left, and he came right in front of you as he was interacting with you. And I just felt like, oh my goodness, here is somebody who really cares about people who are deaf, who really gets what it's like to be deaf. And I was blown away.

Debbie Enstminger: I guess seeing that, hearing recommendations about him, I just felt such a blessing to have him and that gave real peace, knowing that I was in the hands of somebody... I remember the day I went in for surgery, he was doing five surgeries that day. This is somebody I had read online where they recommended find a surgeon who does at least 50 surgeries a year, preferably with most of them being with the type of cochlear implant you're being implanted with.

Richard: But your surgery was very complicated. I understand you had a unique situation.

Debbie Enstminger: Yes. Dr. Bartels was the first person to ever diagnose my hearing loss, because it was a very different hearing loss. Which is one of the reasons why hearing aids didn't work for me, was because instead of a gradual slope on my audiogram, it was more like a cliff. Where I heard, I heard normal, what I didn't hear, there was nothing. So there really wasn't anything for hearing aids to amplify if that makes sense. That's why it got in the way of me hearing.

Debbie Enstminger: Dr. Bartels looked at me. I described what it was. And he said, "Oh, that's Bing Siebenmann dysplasia." He had a younger person in there who he was educating about this, and it was the most fascinating thing, because honestly, I'd had all sorts of experimental tests and everything where doctors would try to determine what this hearing loss was from, and he immediately knew what it was. What he told me was, he said, he had to insert the electrodes... I may be getting the details wrong, but I think it was about 16 millimeters, a little bit deeper. At least a little bit deeper into the cochlear.

Debbie Enstminger: That meant even though I probably could have qualified for getting both at once, he said, "Let's start with just one, because since I have to insert the electrodes deeper into the cochlear, there may be greater risk of dizziness. Let's just do one and let's see how it goes." There was-

Richard: If you have the risk of vertigo- Debbie Enstminger: Yes.

Richard: You must have been scared out of your mind on surgery day.

Debbie Enstminger: Do you know, there was that sense that yes, and it was the most incredible thing. The night before my surgery I woke up at 3:00 in the morning, and I just went and I was spending some time with God, because of course my heart is going, you know? I mean, I had total confidence in my doctor, but you don't know. And they make you sign off, there's all these different things that could possibly happen. And I just happened, in my Bible, to be reading the story of when Jesus heals a little girl, and he says to her, "Talitha cumi, little girl, come." And it's interesting, because it's said in the context of as he's on his way to heal this little girl there's a woman who has been bleeding for over a decade, and it says in there, she spent her money on doctors who couldn't help her. And I'm like, "Oh, I hope I'm like the little girl at the end of the story of that one."

Debbie Enstminger: But it just felt like the Lord was just saying, "Come, I'm with you. I'm taking you this way." There wasn't an assurance that there wouldn't be complications, because sometimes the way God leads is hard, but I had a peace that if there was that he would carry me through. He would help me. But yes, I probably would not be human if there wasn't that sense of some anxiety that you're feeling. And it was so good. I painted that night because painting just helps me process emotions.

Richard: You mentioned your husband. You met him... Obviously you had a hearing loss at the time, and it got worse with time. Talk to me a little bit about how he dealt with your hearing loss.

Debbie Enstminger: Oh, do you know? He's such a gift to me. I mean, he really is. I often say I think it's harder for the person who's married to someone with hearing loss than it is for us who have the hearing loss, because he had to constantly be adapting too. He couldn't call to me from another room. He had to repeat himself. God bless that man. He really tried so hard to keep me involved, to paraphrase when people were saying things. I love his sense of humor, his laugh, because you know, you'll be in the middle of a dinner conversation and somebody will ask you something, and lipreading is really a misnomer. It's not like reading, like reading words on a page. You can only get maximum maybe 30% of the words. It's more like fill in the blank, a very educated guessing game, where context helps. But there are times I'll completely hear wrong. And then, suddenly, the room kind of gets quiet as people look at one another real funny.

Richard: Some people withdraw into isolation because they're afraid to open their mouth and say the wrong thing in a group.

Debbie Enstminger: Yes.

Richard: But not you.

Debbie Enstminger: No.

Richard: You just blurted it right out.

Debbie Enstminger: Well, it's because Jim... He just kept encouraging me. "Keep a sense of humor, babe." You know? Just, "Keep a sense of humor. We can tell them it's not early onset Alzheimer's," you know? And he'd always go to bat for me. "She didn't hear you." Or sometimes he'd say, "Sweetie, what do you think they said?" And I'd say that, and we'd all just roar out laughing because if you can keep a sense of the fun in life instead of taking it personally, you know, you do the best you can.

Richard: You are very strong. Most people take it personally.

Debbie Enstminger: Well, I'm sure there are times, but-

Richard: Now you decide to move forward. You had your operation. How did you choose the company? I'm sure that they must have done what

we call a document dump where they just dump all the manufacturers on your lap and say, "Choose one." How did you go about choosing what you did?

Debbie Enstminger: Do you know, that was one of the hardest things, because the way everything is set up nobody wants to tell you what to do. And I felt so unbelievably alone. Obviously, I ran to the Lord. I was really praying about this. It was interesting, one of the companies sent me a book and I jokingly told my husband, "Anybody who sends me a book gets my business." But then as I started moving forward, I started to feel like maybe that was going to be the best choice for me. Moving forward with that. Just the week before I was going for my scheduled preop appointment, okay? And I just cried out the Lord, and I was like, "God, I just feel so unbelievably alone. Would you please just send me somebody who can help me?"

Debbie Enstminger: It was interesting, because one of the companies had sent me an email, and the person had said, "Hey, if you have any questions just email me back, I'd be so happy to answer them." I sent her an email back, and I get immediate response that that message had gone into her spam folder. I was just like, "Oh, my goodness." Then I just happened to get another email that day from Cochlear America, and they told me that there was going to be a meeting in Rome, Georgia, on the exact day of my... You know, coming up in Rome, Georgia. That's eight hours away from me. I'm like, "How did I get on this list?"

Debbie Enstminger: But there was a name of a contact person, so I sent her an email, and I was like, "Look, is there anybody closer to me who I could possibly meet with to talk about this?" Because at that point Cochlear America had just come out with the N7, and I was like, "I would love to meet somebody who got an N7, just to talk with them, to hear about what it's like. I think it would just help me feel so much better."

Debbie Enstminger: She immediately emails me back, says, "I would be glad to meet with you," and she sent me the name of this wonderful gentleman named Richard Pocker. That next day, we met at Starbucks, and that was a huge game-changer. To be able to meet with somebody. Because, you know, what's hard is the way this is all set up between surgeons and audiologists, and everybody, there is a business side to it. It's hard to get people to give you a clear answer. "Well, I really think you should do this one, or that." It needs to be your decision, and that's why I'm so thankful there's things like-

Richard: That's part of the medical profession- Debbie Enstminger: Oh, it is.

Richard: ... and the FDA rules, that's just the way it is.

Debbie Enstminger: Yeah.

Richard: They're not supposed to recommend. Activation day. You get turned on. What did you hear?

Debbie Enstminger: Oh, goodness. Well, that was where I was so very, very thankful that I had received an email that morning telling me, where you had shared about your experience that morning with me, just that when you were activated, you didn't hear immediately. What I loved about that, and so appreciated about getting that email, when I went in for activation, my expectations were lower.

Debbie Enstminger: I was so glad because I was like, "I do not want anybody videotaping this. I don't want the pressure." You know what I'm saying? Of being watched because I don't know what it's going to be like. Because it could have been that I regained voice recognition right away. It could have been that I just didn't... I heard bells and whistles or something. I could have just been that I heard sensations or something. I wasn't sure what to expect.

Debbie Enstminger: It was interesting, because when Dr. Vicky Moore, when she did the first test, and that's not one where you're hearing at all, I didn't realize it at the time, but she said my auditory nerves were non-responsive. And one of the representatives from Cochlear America was present when I was being activated, and she said, "I don't know if you saw, but I looked back at Katie Figueroa and I thought, "Uh oh." But then when she started piping in sound, it felt like being plopped into the middle of a Looney Tunes cartoon. I was hearing bells and whistles, pops, and jingles, and it was so crazy.

Debbie Enstminger: Vicky asked me a question and I answered, and it was the wildest thing, because I opened my mouth and bells, and whistles are coming out of my mouth. I thought, "I'm never going to talk again."

Richard: How long did it take for the sounds to normalize? I know everybody's different. What was your experience?"

Debbie Enstminger: It was the most amazing thing. As we're sitting there in that first audiology appointment, the activation was a little over an hour and a half long. Towards the end of the activation appointment, suddenly, I started realizing, "Wait a minute, those bells, those whistles," started taking shape as words. I was like, "Wait a minute, I think that's a word. That is a word." By the end of the appointment, I was understanding my husband. Now, he sounded like a robot.

Richard: That is essentially what Jim sounds like.

Debbie Enstminger: But it was the most amazing thing. I was like, "I'm hearing what you're saying." I was understanding it. And as we drove home, we're driving home in the car, and I had downloaded the Angel Sounds app which is an app that can help you practice. So as my first time ever doing it, I scored 75% on it. Now, some of it may have been educated guessing, but I was like, "This is amazing." We get home and my husband says, "Deb, go into the other room," because with the N7 the iPhone streams directly in now. And he goes, "Let's just see how it works."

Debbie Enstminger: He went into the other side of the house, and he called me, and the first thing I ever heard on the phone was my husband saying, "I love you."

Richard: Aw. That's so nice. You know, that brings us back two or three steps to all the years you didn't have hearing, how did you deal with the phone? You just couldn't use a phone, obviously?

Debbie Enstminger: You know, it was so funny. In the beginning... This is 14 years ago. I had a little flip phone, and what I would do is, the University of South Florida, where I was on campus at the time, I'd go to meet with students, and they'd be up in their dorms. I would dial them, and I'd say, "Hey, I'm downstairs." If they said anything other than, "I'll be right down," which I figured how that would go, I would have to grab hold of a student who happened to be walking by and say, "Excuse me, could you please tell me what they're saying?"

Richard: That's another adaptation, which brings us to story, what happens if you needed 911? If you needed help and you were deaf and you couldn't use the phone? Did you ever have an incident where you were helpless?

Debbie Enstminger: Yes. I had been speaking at a women's retreat. There was a lot of cleaning up and everything to do, and so almost everybody had left. And I went outside, and my car wouldn't start. I had my phone, and this is before cochlear implant, and I'm calling AAA. And I'm saying into my phone, "Okay, I can't tell if anybody's picked up, and I'm here, but I'm going to read you, this is my name, and this is my AAA number, and this is my location, would you please come? And just in case you hadn't picked up yet when I started, I'm going to repeat the information." I repeated it about three times, and then I just hung up and was just waiting. Thankfully, there was one woman who was still there, and she came over.

Debbie Enstminger: At that point, I was telling her about what was happening, because the battery had died in my car. And she said, "Well, let me just call AAA." She dials the number for AAA, and this is right after Hurricane Irma, and she goes, "Oh, there's no phone service." I had just been sitting there-

Richard: There are other people I've interviewed and that's the key question I have is about how did you deal with an emergency? Because one of the things that we like to talk about is the motivation for getting a cochlear implant, that you're no longer dependent on others to help you. You use the phone today without hesitation?

Debbie Enstminger: Oh, now, it's the most wonderful thing. In fact, it expanded my work even more, because now I coach using Zoom. I can coach people online. I'm able to coach people on the other side of the world.

Richard: Which is great. Were there other things that you had changed in your life after you got a CI? After you got a cochlear implant, what other changes can you talk about?

Debbie Enstminger: Oh, my goodness, there are so many things. You know, it's funny, you don't realize, I don't think, the things that you're missing. It was interesting, because a television station wanted to do an interview with me, and one of the students that I met with. It was the most fascinating thing, because they're asking her, because she met with me before cochlear implants for a year and a half, and then met with me for half a year afterwards, and so they were like, "What was the difference before and after?"

Debbie Enstminger: She said, "Well, you know, before I just kind of told her the bare bones of things because I knew she was working so hard to understand. But now I can share so much more of life in so much more detail." And I was like, "I didn't know that people weren't telling me everything they wanted to tell me." I told my husband that and he goes, "Oh yeah, that's true for me too." And it is the most wonderful thing to be sharing so much more of life with my husband, able to hear what he has to say. When it was dark, I could never read his lips. Now I can hear everything that he wants to say. It's the most amazing gift just to be able to do that.

Debbie Enstminger: I'm a cyclist. I love biking. I honestly think my guardian angel's going to be so happy when I make it to heaven so they can get a vacation, because when you're hearing impaired, there have been so many times I've almost been hit, because you don't get the feedback of hearing if a car happens to be coming close or anything. It is the most amazing thing now to be able to bike wearing cochlear implants and to get that feedback. I can't even begin to tell- Richard: It's true, it's true.

Debbie Enstminger: ... you how many times it's probably saved my life.

Richard: I was almost run over by a fire engine in New York City. Never heard it coming.

Debbie Enstminger: No.

Richard: I know how that goes.

Debbie Enstminger: Yes.

Richard: Let me ask you another question. You have the Nucleus 7, and now you're bilateral. You got the second- Debbie Enstminger: Yes. Yes.

Richard: ... one six months or a year later. Are there features of the N7 you like in particular? Number one, and number two, are there features you would like to see in the future?

Debbie Enstminger: Do you know something? The fact that the N7 streams the iPhone right into my head is the most amazing gift. It is such a blessing to be able to do that. I'm tech challenged and so having to have an intermediary between the phone and my head would be hard. But it's the most incredible thing, the way it just streams right in. The clarity is just superb.

Richard: What about music? Do you listen to music?

Debbie Enstminger: I do. I play the guitar. And that has taken more. It's been a longer process. And I think that's one of the things... It's interesting. I think because I had to work so hard to hear without a cochlear implant, because I had that pressing in, that adaptability constantly coming in there trying to figure out, how am I going to do this? Has really made me put in my all, 100%. What is it going to take to keep developing my hearing? Because it's so much about your brain. It saddens me. I'll meet people who just don't keep trying and keep growing, and it's been amazing how much my ability has grown. The more I listen, the better results I'm getting, and the better I'm hearing. When I first started playing my guitar, it sounded horrible.

Richard: Everybody said that.

Debbie Enstminger: I was like, "Oh my gosh." Richard: What about now?

Debbie Enstminger: Oh, it's amazing, because with finger picking... What happened was I think chords were overwhelming the brain. Same thing with the piano. There is nothing like sitting down to a piano and hearing the clarity of the individual notes. Do you know what I'm saying? When I first started out, the singers that I would hear, I thought if they could hear themselves through my ears they would never sing again. It was so bad.

Debbie Enstminger: When I was just in Colorado, one of my nieces has been taking voice lessons, and she sang to me this precious, precious hymn. And she sang this hymn to me, and tears were streaming down my face because her voice sounded so beautiful. This has been such a gift from the Lord that I never even imagined it could get so good.

Richard: That's fantastic. I have one last question for you. I know you traveled a lot in your work. How did you deal with airports before when you were deaf?

Debbie Enstminger: So, when I'm stateside, I always loved to travel Southwest Airlines because they let me board first. And that is such a gift, because one time I was traveling another airline that didn't allow that, and they suddenly announced over the intercom that the gate had changed. What happens is when you travel, and I'm on high alert the whole time, I am constantly looking for clues. I can't just sit back and read a book or something. I'm constantly... And I happened to notice a significant number of people went from one gate to another gate. I walked up to the front... And this is what's bad. I had told them, "I'm hearing impaired, can you let me know if there's a change," and they didn't. I walked up to the front and said, "Excuse me, I happened to notice a lot of people just moved," and they said, "Oh yes, that flight has changed to the other end of the airport." I would have completely missed.

Debbie Enstminger: There have been a couple times I've almost missed my flight, and thankfully it's never happened, but that's one of the reasons why I'm just so thankful that Southwest lets me pre-board. I tell them I'm deaf, they go out of their way for me. When I travel internationally, I try to ask people around me. I don't know, it's something like, when you're traveling you can kind of look and scope out, who seems friendly? And you'll just start talking to people, and I'll say, "I am deaf." Again, it's that not letting fear or pride shut me down but asking for help. And I'll just ask somebody.

Debbie Enstminger: I remember the first time I was traveling to the Middle East, there was a gentleman, he was so wonderful. He said, "I will watch out for you as if you were my daughter." And he... What's just amazing, through the entire process, he just walked me right through.

Richard: But since you've gotten your cochlear implants, are the sound systems in the airport any better?

Debbie Enstminger: Yes. That is the most amazing thing, because here's the deal. With cochlear implants, again, they're not exactly like your ear would be if you had that. So, if I'm in conversation with somebody, I may be focusing in on the person and not hear that. But you know what? Even if I could hear normally, I'm the type of person who doesn't tend to focus on things out there anyways. I probably do better with flights because I'm aware I need to be paying more attention.

Debbie Enstminger: But no, it's amazing to hear the announcements, to do that. But I will say it's funny because one of the things I most feared was losing my residual hearing. And even at zero there was probably still a little bit that I could still hear. Now, I'm on a plane and there's a screaming baby next to me, I turn my processors off, and it is the most wonderful flight. I say people probably wish they could buy these.

Richard: You know, it's true about the residual hearing, because there was a woman I helped in Louisiana, and she had zero on one side, 4% on the other. And it took her almost two years to decide to move ahead. She was afraid of losing the 4%.

Debbie Enstminger: Yeah.

Richard: It's not an uncommon fear. I have one last question. I'm going to let you go.

Debbie Enstminger: Yes.

Richard: What's your goal now that you have your hearing back? What are you going to do differently?

Debbie Enstminger: Do you know, it's interesting. I love my job, so it's not like I'm going to be changing anything else that I'm doing. I think one of the things that's on my heart is to really come alongside and encourage people... Because this is what's really fascinating. There was one day when I was deaf and I was going to campus, and it was like... This was when I had lost all my hearing. And I was like, "Lord, I don't even know, am I even going to be able to do any good?" Because there were some people I just could not understand.

Debbie Enstminger: And I just felt like he said, "Just go and do what you can." And showing up. And the first student I ran into on campus was deaf. She was severely hearing impaired, and she had been experiencing a progressive loss, and was down about it. It was the most amazing thing, orchestrated by Him, but it is amazing with students, we all have things we go through that are hard in life, and I love being able to just encourage people, lean in. Don't pull back. Keep giving it your all. And so being available to just really encourage people to trust the Lord with their circumstances, to keep crying out to Him for ideas, to adapt, and to make the most of it because my heart's desire is I want to see everybody possible live life to the full, as much as they can. I just think how Jesus said, "I have come, they may have life and have it to the full." I want to see that. I want to see people, no matter what their circumstances, no matter what hard things come their way in life, experience all the best that the Lord has for them.

Richard: You're a remarkable person. I thank you so much for your time.

Debbie Enstminger: Oh, thank you, Richard.

CHAPTER 8 SUE WOLFE SMITH

SIMULTANEOUS BILATERAL COCHLEAR IMPLANT SURGERY. ONE SURGERY. ONE REHABILITATION.

As she describes it, Sue had a lifelong progressive moderate to profound sensorineural hearing loss in both ears.

Wearing hearing aids from the age of eight, she struggled but used many of the compensation tricks that are familiar to those of us with a hearing loss.

But she went beyond what we may have done, and her story would take hours and provide an encyclopedia of useful tips.

My interest was to have her focus on music, a topic of major interest to many candidates. Her involvement with music and being married to a musician, meant that as her hearing loss progressed, her world was shrinking.

Sue received bilateral cochlear implant surgery and was activated with two Cochlear Nucleus 7s in 2018.

She talks about her experience with music both pre and post activation.

Richard: Sue Wolfe Smith was introduced to me over two years ago when she was first investigating cochlear implants. Her severe hearing loss, which she describes in her interview, was at an impasse. As we communicated over the weeks, it became obvious to me that music played a huge part in Sue's life and her questions were often oriented to that aspect of cochlear implants. While all cochlear implants are first and foremost concerned with speech comprehension, I talked about my own experiences with hearing music again for the first time in 35 years, and like me, Sue was qualified for bilateral surgery. And like me, she was scared to proceed. In the end, she did get bilateral cochlear implants. She received two Cochlear Nucleus 7s. I wanted her to share her experiences with hearing music again. It's a question that is of primary importance to many, many candidates for cochlear implants.

Sue Wolfe Smith: I began having difficulty with my hearing when I was eight years old. A routine school testing discovered a deficiency, so they sent me to a specialized audiologist who tested me further, and they determined that I needed a hearing aid in my left ear. I started wearing a hearing aid in my left ear at that age. I got a second hearing aid when I was 14. I have sensorineural loss, and they didn't have any explanation for it, so it was kind of a mystery to all of us. There's no hereditary hearing loss in my family. It's just one of those things. It may have been caused by a childhood illness, who knows? But anyways, it was moderate to severe at that age, and it just gradually progressed over my lifetime, worse, and I eventually lost most of my high frequencies within the last probably 15 to 20 years. I'm 58 now. I got a second hearing aid at the age of 14. Once I had that, it was better, but it was still always a struggle to understand speech.

Richard: Right.

Sue Wolf Smith: So, I was totally reliant on lip reading.

Richard: You depended on lip reading in high school and college. What kinds of support did you get there?

Sue Wolfe Smith: Well, it was just basically the hearing AIDS, you know. I went and got my hearing tested at the Santa Fe School for the Deaf, but as far as school, I just met your regular public schools. I learned to talk to my teachers about seating me at the front where I could hear better and see them, and I learned that I had to be proactive and ask questions to get the information that I missed, because I missed a lot. Somehow I managed to get the information I needed from reading and talking to the teacher, talking to my co-students, that sort of thing.

Richard: You were mainstreamed. Your parents never considered a school for deaf or hard of hearing or anything?

Sue Wolfe Smith: I don't think they seriously considered it. I think they felt that my loss was mild enough and that I had the support of the teachers and staff that I would do okay in a public-school setting. It wasn't total deafness, you know, it was just a mild loss. I was able to function just fine in a public-school setting.

Richard: Your severe loss really occurred after college, in other words?

Sue Wolfe Smith: I always had severe loss at higher frequencies than at low frequency. I did have good low-frequency residual, but it did gradually get worse. It was probably around college, maybe 10 years after, that it really started taking a nosedive over that time. Yeah.

Richard: Okay. You got out of college, and you had to find a job because you weren't always in the picture framing business. What was your career like?

Sue Wolfe Smith: Well, I didn't go straight into my career. I went back to graduate school, but for two years in between college and grad school, I was doing odd jobs, renovation and remodeling, landscaping, restaurant work, that sort of thing. Then I moved to Arizona and went back to school for museum work, so that was really my focus was anthropology and museum studies, both as an undergraduate and as a graduate. But then I got married. So, I didn't really finish the master's degree, but that's just me. That's another story.

Richard: That didn't have to deal with your hearing loss?

Sue Wolfe Smith: No, not really. I think I did well, overall, as a student because I knew to be proactive and ask for the information that I missed, but I still felt like I missed quite a bit during those days because you can't get everything. You're only limited to what you can see, read, and lip read and so it's kind of difficult. But I managed to get through it well. There wasn't work available in that field. That's kind of how I got into the printing business, because we got married and then I moved back to Kansas with my husband, and I had to find a job. This was a time when the humanities were taking a dive, and nobody was hiring in the museum field unless you volunteered first. I needed a paying job and I ended up in the frame shop at Michael's stores. That's how I started framing.

Richard: You learned at Michael's. Everybody must start somewhere.

Sue Wolfe Smith: Yes, I did. You didn't know that?

Richard: What about, talk to me about how you dealt with the customers with your hearing loss.

Sue Wolfe Smith: Well, I am pretty much very, again, lip reading reliant. I could hear with my hearing aids. I had two hearing aids, right? And I could hear them talking to me, but I couldn't understand them unless I could see them. For the most part, I was able to function just fine on the counter, as long as I could deal one on one, I could not use the phone well. I could not understand the PA system at Michael's stores, but there were enough other framers that I had support there to fill in those blanks, if needed. I went into management at those shops, and I did just fine. The phone was one thing I couldn't do, pretty much.

Richard: That's important, our not being able to use the phone. Did other people make the calls for you?

Sue Wolfe Smith: Yes, other people made and took calls. I attempted to take calls early on, but after a couple of years, I just couldn't understand a word being said to me. It was gibberish, so I gave it up. I just stopped using the phone.

Richard: That's interesting, because other people I've interviewed said that they had to leave their careers because they could not use the phone, or they could not deal with clients because the clients expect them to be fully functional. You found the same thing?

Sue Wolfe Smith: It was a disadvantage, and it's even more so of a disadvantage when I left Michael's and opened my own shop, but I have always been able to work around it. Sometimes you must rely on the good in people to help you out, and I think that's a large part of how I got through all of that, because it was just so hard not being able to communicate by phone. It's such a thing that's taken for granted, but then came faxing and emailing and all these messaging technologies came up, and that just helped me pick up the ball and run with it. People are willing to work with you. Sometimes I have to wonder, though, how much business I lost because I couldn't hear or use the phone.

Richard: That's a very interesting point, very interesting point.

Sue Wolfe Smith: I can tell you more about how I've coped at my own business. Even though I don't use assistive technology, I have an answering machine that says I'm hearing impaired, leave a message. Originally it said leave a message, fax, or email and gave an email address. I managed okay that way, but you've got to wonder how many people would call that machine, get that message, and just hang up. So that was always haunting me.

Richard: That's an excellent point.

Sue Wolfe Smith: Yeah.

Richard: You don't know what you're missing when you have a hearing loss. That's a point we make repeatedly. Well, let me ask you about support you got from your family and your friends and your church. Did they all stick by you? Did anybody disappoint you?

Sue Wolfe Smith: Oh yes, very much so. Yes. Just everyone, family, friends, the schools for my children, kids, everyone knew about my hearing impairment because I made it known to them. I think it's very important for this sort of disability. You must communicate with people about it. I can understand that it's easy to withdraw and be insecure and shy about it, but you must let them know that you have to communicate this way, and most of the time they will.

Richard: Okay. I wanted to interview you, especially, because of your involvement with music. A lot of people who are candidates or recipients struggle with music, but you seem to have a unique perspective, so I wish you would talk about that for a few minutes. The change from hearing aids to cochlear implants.

Sue Wolfe Smith: I've got to say, it sounds pretty darn good. Right off, I have a background in music. I lived in the bass line for a long time because of the high frequency loss that I had, and as those high frequencies went away, my husband is a musician, so I'm exposed to music on a regular basis, and I grew up with music, so that's a big part of my life. With hearing aids, it gradually became less and less of the melody, the high instrumentals, the upper register sounds began to disappear, which was very distressing because my husband would sing a song, he'd been singing for 20 years, and all of a sudden I didn't recognize it because I don't hear his part of it anymore.

Sue Wolfe Smith: So that was very distressing with hearing aids. By the time I got to cochlear implants, I agonized over that decision to go bilateral, because I knew it was going to change and I knew it wasn't going to sound as good, but I also knew from talking to other people, that it's possible to rehabilitate it to where it sounds pretty good, which it does. My experience with that switch is that before I didn't have the highs, I was still missing half the music, whereas after, the lows go away, which we all know. The bass goes away because the electrode array doesn't extend all the way into the cochlea, and you're also being inundated with all of this high sound that you haven't had, either you haven't ever had, or you haven't had it for a very long time.

Sue Wolfe Smith: To me, it seems like early on with the cochlear implants, it was distorted. It was just overwhelmingly vocals and high instrumentals, and I couldn't understand the lyrics. I've never been able to understand lyrics, ever. Gradually, with rehabilitation, it got to a point where I'm getting the mid-range and the lower registers back. They're there. I can hear them. They're just hard to hear, and they're not predominant anymore. It's like swapping the bass for the treble. On the other hand, I'm hearing stuff I've never heard in music. I'm able to discriminate instruments, now. I can hear lyrics more and more. I'm hearing crystal clear lyrics, which is unheard of for me. It's just an amazing process, but it takes work. It takes listening, listening, listening to the same stuff over and over and over again.

Richard: That's what I think candidates want to know. Now, you've been implanted now how long?

Sue Wolfe Smith: I've been activated for almost 20 months now.

Richard: 20 months?

Sue Wolfe Smith: I have 20 months, yeah.

Richard: Right, so 20 months, you've gotten most of the music back, but it's improving all the time?

Sue Wolfe Smith: Oh, most definitely. Now, there's qualities to the music that are still lacking. It's not your natural hearing, obviously. But it's pretty darn good. I find myself struggling to find the right terms to describe what I'm experiencing or not experiencing, as it may be. But sometimes it seems a little toneless. I also find that I'm getting that back, that feeling of tonality and harmony. On one hand I hear all this stuff great, and it still moves me. I still love it. It's still music. I'm so happy about that.

Richard: It's interesting when you say you can't find the terms. It always brings me back to that scene in the movie of Children of a Lesser God when she was deaf and he had hearing, and he's trying to describe music to her. He couldn't find the terms.

Sue Wolfe Smith: I haven't seen that movie. I need to see that. But yeah, that's exactly right. It's just a richness that natural hearing has. I've experienced that. However, what I get now, these are sounds that I really have never heard on this level, and even though the bass has fallen into the background more, that's where it's supposed to be. The bass shouldn't be the first thing that you hear about a piece. The other thing I've noticed is that different music sounds different. Some things sound better than others. That's going to be the rule no matter what, but a lot has to do with personal preference, too.

Sue Wolfe Smith: This is hard to convey sometimes. I would just like to say that, given focused rehabilitation with pitch apps, it could probably continue to improve. I feel like I am continuing to improve over this time. I haven't reached my full potential with music yet. I can feel that it gets better the more I do with it. I'm listening to an album that I've never heard. I know maybe one or two songs from long ago. Van Morrison is who I'm listening to right now, and I know almost all the songs on that, just listening to it now. I needed a little help looking at lyrics and stuff, but just focusing on repetition really helps a lot, and you start hearing things that you didn't hear.

Sue Wolfe Smith: It helps me to have a musician husband sitting next to me in the car saying, "Can you hear that organ?" Or "That's a harmonica." Sometimes I'll need help. Say, "That sounds like a trumpet. Is that a trumpet?" "Nope, it's a sax." I'd go back and I listened to it again. Then, "Oh yeah, that's a sax. I can hear that little quality of sound that a saxophone has." It's just this constant process of identifying and then going back again, identify then go back and listen to it again, and your brain just picks it up that way. It's crazy.

Richard: It's fabulous.

Sue Wolfe Smith: It's amazing.

Richard: That is fabulous.

Sue Wolfe Smith: Yeah, I'm totally blown away. I'm happy with that outcome. It will never be exactly the same. I accept that. I'm okay with that because I gained a lot. You know, I've lost a lot, but I also gained a lot, so I'm happy. It's a balance. It's something I can always work on. Yes.

Richard: Fabulous results, fabulous results. So, as long as you had Greg with you to help you with the music, you made faster progress than most people would make with music. And better results, probably.

Sue Wolfe Smith: Well, and it didn't sound good at first. I'm just like everyone else. I'm "This sounds awful." I listened to my favorite James Taylor CD, and I was just, "Oh man, this sounds horrible." At the very beginning, okay? Honestly, Richard. I was just, "Oh God, what have I gotten myself into?" I had a stereo system in my shop with speakers. Greg has a PA system in here for his music, and I played James Taylor's

Hourglass, which was my therapy CD before CIs. I mean, I'd listen to that over and over again. I have a habit of loving a CD and then just putting it on a loop and listening to it repeatedly. It drives my husband nuts. But he likes these guys, too.

Richard: Yeah, that's a great way. I love that. I love that.

Sue Wolfe Smith: That CD, the James Taylor CD, was my benchmark because I listened to that and it was a relatively new one, so I didn't know the higher parts of that CD very well because I wasn't hearing them. When I put it in the stereo system at the shop right after my activation, it was like, "Oh my God, this sounds horrible." I could not recognize the songs at all, and it was distressing. But I thought, "Okay, Richard said it sounds good. Richard said it sounds good." Just keep listening and you're hearing memory starts to kick in, and then the more you listen, you remember the song, you remember how it goes, and suddenly, you're hearing it again.

Sue Wolfe Smith: It takes a while. I spent probably a couple of months listening to that one CD, but there were some others that I pulled in. My thing was to go through the CDs and see what sounded good that I remembered and listen to those. And that's what I did. Dan Fogelberg was the other one. Dan Fogelberg and James Taylor. And you know what? James started to sound pretty good after a while. It was just like a whole new dimension on these songs. It was neat in that way. Even though it may not be perfect music hearing, it's still, it's all this stuff. All these high rickety percussion sounds and oh my gosh, things that had gone away had come back. It's kind of a mixed experience. You know?

Richard: That's right, yeah. Well, you know, when we first met through social media and you were trying to find reasons to move forward and we talked about it many times, and because you and I are unique that we both had bilateral surgery. Now from your point of view, why did you decide to go bilateral in the one operation?

Sue Wolfe Smith: Well, you were instrumental in that decision, but my thinking was, and I had read enough studies about the benefits and advantages of binaural hearing and the things that your brain does with two ears that I can't do with just one. That was one reason. Secondly, I was given that option by my surgeon, and I'm like, "I'm being given a gift here. I have a choice." Both of my ears are equally bad by that time. The other thing was my hearing aids were old. They needed to be replaced, one had cracked out, just been repaired. Having a CI in one ear and an old hearing aid in the other ear really wasn't going to do me that much good, and I couldn't afford a brand-new hearing aid. So that was the practical economical aspect of it. And then of course there's one surgery, one recovery, one rehab. Your ears are rehabbing together. Your brain has both ears working at the same time. It just made sense to me.

Richard: That does make sense. And you know that one of the issues that comes up on social media all the time is that the activation day, the expectations now are very, very high because they see videos just like yours where you're understanding speech at the turn on. But it's unique. How did you feel on activation day? Everybody's seeing your video.

Sue Wolfe Smith: Oh God, I feel so guilty, because I know that so many people don't get that, and so many people struggle for months after activation just to hear a word. I totally feel blessed with that. I'm just so lucky that that's how it went for me. On the other hand, though, what's interesting about that is that my ears aren't the same. One ear is significantly worse than the other ear. So that's kind of an interesting thing, because if I had chosen the worst ear, it might have been a whole other trip. You know, I might not have gone bilateral. But as it was, I got booth ears activated, and the video was with my right ear, and that was the first ear she turned on. My right ear is my stronger ear. It hears much more clarity and speech. It's just amazing how clear it was right off the bat.

Sue Wolfe Smith: And I think after the left year was activated, I realized what a difference there was between them. The two ears together hear almost perfectly. It's great. The left ear still lags. It's one thing about going bilateral at the same time eliminates is any question of which ear is better, you know. I will always push for implanting the better ear, if your ears are more or less the same if you want to do one at a time, because that ear probably has better stimulation history. My right ear was always my better ear as a kid. You know, my left ear was always worse. Even though they were about the same just before I got implanted, my right ear is so much better. I don't know if that's because of my ears, I don't know if it's because of my surgeon being right-handed or left-handed, I don't know if it's because a resident did my left ear? They told me that wasn't the case. I had to ask.

Richard: Now you activated, you're guilty that you did so well, and my next question to you is how has your cochlear implant changed your life? Is it for better or worse, changes at work, with family, with your friends?

Sue Wolfe Smith: It is so much better. My world has opened wide. I am still afraid of the phone, but I am gradually overcoming that and that's a psychological thing. I can understand speech perfectly through the iPhone. The streaming's amazing. Everyday life, it's so much easier to deal with people in general. I don't have to struggle to watch every moment to understand what's being said to me. I had to feel left out in a group. I really don't have to say I can't use the phone, even though I'm still doing that. I'm realizing that I can understand pretty good. And I'm telling you, this is something I've never had. It is just the most amazing experience, and I can't thank people who work on this technology enough. The surgeons, the audiologists, Cochlear Americas. I'm telling you, it's just amazing. I just can't say any more than that. It's been amazing being able to communicate with people with so much less effort.

Richard: Well, you know, that's a very interesting question as well about obviously you don't have any regrets. I haven't heard one yet. Are there any features you like in particular? You're wearing the Nucleus 7, but are there any features you like, or features you'd like to see in the future?

Sue Wolfe Smith: Well, I totally love the ability to stream from my phone. That's an awesome feature. I maybe don't use it as much as I should, but it sure is neat. Another thing about that, too, is that streamed music sounds different from music that you listen to in the open sound field, like in a room or in a car. It kind of gives my brain the best of both worlds. Really, the only complaints that I have are how the coil gets tangled up in my hair, and then the processor doesn't sit on my ear so well sometimes. You know, it's still stuff like that. Minor inconveniences, compared to the joy that I get just being able to hear. I don't care about the rest of that stuff.

Sue Wolfe Smith: It's just so fantastic to go outside and hear crickets and cicadas and frogs and all these sounds that I knew as a kid. It takes me straight back. I think it's still a little rough around the edges sometimes, but that really is my only complaint. That's just something I've accepted. It does bother me that it's not perfect. Because I can hear it pretty darn good.

Richard: Well, now that you have your hearing back, are there any goals you have for the future, anything you would do differently now?

Sue Wolfe Smith: I haven't really thought along those lines, but you know, it occurred to me I could go back to school. I mean, I could go back to school even if I couldn't hear, but that's just having learned to cope all my life. Right now, I'm well entrenched in my business, and I don't really have anything I'd rather be doing at this point, which would be relevant to my improved hearing. I'm just saying that it's so much easier. You know, I've taken on something I would never have done before I had these. I am on the board of my local historical society museum. I have been for 20 years. I've always muddled through the meetings and again, missed so much.

Sue Wolfe Smith: Well, shortly after I was activated and hearing all this amazing stuff, our board president decided he was going to resign and relocate, and so we had to find a new board president. Yep. You guessed it. They nominated me, and I'm just going, "Can I really do this? Yes, you can do this Sue. You can run a meeting." It was hard for me to say, "Okay, sure, I'll do it." I'm still a little uncomfortable. It's only been a couple of months, so I'm president of the board of trustees at the Clearwater Historical Museum, too. But you know, things like that, I'm no longer terrified to do them. I'm no longer afraid to take on something like that just because I can't hear, because I can hear. Little things in life have just gotten so much easier.

Richard: That's the major thing in life, not a minor thing. All right, my last question for you is do you have advice for others who might be sitting on the fence?

Sue Wolfe Smith: Just do it. I know there are risks involved, but the repercussions of not doing it are worse. I've seen how having this wonderful hearing, even though it takes a while for some people, can help you cope with things that happen to you and to your loved ones. If you can advocate for other people, that's one thing you can do. If you don't do this, you're going to suffer. You're still going to be struggling to understand. You're still going to be missing out on life. There're just so many things that you could accomplish with improved hearing. I think that the risks, even though they're there, the surgical techniques have improved, the technology has improved. You really have a much better chance of gaining something from it than if you don't do it, you won't gain a thing. It's just going to get worse. That's why I would say, just do it. If you're qualified and you're struggling and feeling socially isolated, you really don't have much to lose, and you have everything to gain.

Richard: Okay. That's true. I would basically say, if you do nothing, nothing will improve. Sue, I really appreciate your time.

CHAPTER 9 JANET FOX PART 1

CONSIDERING GOING FOR THE SECOND SIDE

I met Janet just after she received a cochlear implant three years ago. There was a genetic component to her hearing loss. Her brother received a cochlear implant before she did.

She is an intrepid personality who refused to give up even as she was struggling to get the best results.

Activated with a Cochlear Nucleus 6 and wearing a ReSound hearing aid in the other ear, her bimodal hearing was never optimal. I believed at the time; she would eventually opt to get a second cochlear implant.

As her hearing in the HA side declined, she was ready.

I asked her to sit down with me to talk about her experiences and her decision to go bilateral.

She also shares her experience with tinnitus and how receiving the first cochlear implant influenced it.

Note: This interview was in two parts. There is a follow up after activation of her second side.

Richard: Let me ask you a little bit about your hearing loss. What caused it? Do you have any idea?

Janet Fox: Well, I know I have noise damage, and its part hereditary. I worked with power tools, so I had a lot of loud noises. And at the time, they didn't have any noise stoppers. And loud music. But I think most of its hereditary.

Richard: When did you start to wear hearing aids? At what age were you then?

Janet Fox: I was in my forties. I guess about 20 years ago. And I was at work and people were starting to tell me, "Janet, you can't hear." Richard: Wow.

Janet Fox: Yeah, I'm like, "I'm fine. I'm good, really." But then I started to notice that I kept saying, "What?" a lot.

Richard: What did you then? What happened after that?

Janet Fox: Well, I was a counselor, so I was dealing with people. My boss told me, "Janet, you have to get hearing aids." Well, I wanted to keep my job, so I got one hearing aid and it helped. I could understand people, my clients could talk to me, I could hear them. I guess about five years later I couldn't hear as well.

Richard: It was progressive. It got worse progressively.

Janet Fox: Yeah. It was slowly getting worse.

Richard: You have a brother who also had a hearing problem, so it was hereditary.

Janet Fox: Hereditary. My father had a hearing problem, my cousin has a hearing problem.

Richard: It was all there before.

Janet Fox: Yeah.

Richard: Okay. Your boss was supportive?

Janet Fox: Oh yeah.

Richard: Your clients were there. But eventually one day you realized...

Janet Fox: I didn't hear them. And that's not really conducive to counseling.

Richard: No, not at all. So how did you deal with the telephone? What was going on there?

Janet Fox: I just said, "What?" A lot. And "Could you speak up, please?"

Janet Fox: But basically, I said, "What?" A lot.

Richard: Tell me about the day you realized you had to stop. How did you feel that day? You realized at some point you couldn't do the job anymore. How did you feel that day?

Janet Fox: How did I feel? Well, it was kind of like okay, this is what you got to do. I just did what I had to do. I got angry because I really didn't want to not hear. And I didn't want hearing aids. And it was a vanity thing, too. I really didn't want them.

Janet Fox: But I had a coworker and he had two hearing aids, and he seemed to hear where everything fine, you know? I said, "Okay, this is what

I have to do."

Richard: That was the motivation to move forward, was the coworker?

Janet Fox: Yeah.

Richard: All right. So that was a great influence to get your hearing aids, and your hearing continued to deteriorate. At what point did you consider a cochlear implant?

Janet Fox: After I retired and we moved to Florida, that's when I got my second hearing aid. And after about five years of being here I guess, maybe four years, they weren't working anymore. My brother just got a cochlear implant you know, and I'm looking at him like, "You're crazy," you know? Yeah. "You're out of your mind. Why are you doing this?"

Janet Fox: And I watched him go through the process, and after his surgery, he got activated. He could hear. I mean, my brother was ... I can't say he was worse, whatever you want to say. His hearing was more ...

Richard: Profound loss?

Janet Fox: Yeah.

Richard: Okay.

Janet Fox: And then my husband kept saying, Janet, your hearing's getting worse. So, I decided maybe this is what I need to do.

Richard: What did you do then? What steps did you take at that point?

Janet Fox: Well, we have a friend in New York who wears two hearing aids, and he recommended somebody to me to go see in New York. It turns out that that doctor wasn't in New York anymore, but he was down here in Florida.

Richard: Who was that?

Janet Fox: Dr. Wazen. He came from New York, from Columbia Presbyterian, which is one of the best hospitals in New York. I went to see Dr. Wazen, and I said, "I want a cochlear." Richard: Okay.

Janet Fox: He said, "It's not that simple." I said, "What? I'm deaf. I can't hear anything." He said, "We got to do testing." It didn't take them too long to determine. It's like really, really needed one. And what is it besides cochlear? There's something else.

Richard: BAHA.

Janet Fox: Yeah, it wasn't good for me.

Richard: No. BAHA was not going to work for you. You needed a cochlear implant.

Janet Fox: Right.

Janet Fox: Well, he determined that. And I said, "Okay, let's go through with it." And we did.

Janet Fox: And when they activated me, I was in shock.

Richard: Tell me about the activation day. What was it like?

Janet Fox: I was in shock. I was like, wait a minute, this can't be right. You know, because everybody sounded like R2-D2, very mechanical. I was like on the verge of tears. I can't live with this. I really can't. But it got better.

Richard: How long did it take for it to sound a little better for you?

Janet Fox: Not long. A couple months.

Richard: Wow!

Janet Fox: But then I got a sinus infection. And I don't know what it did, but it was never the same again. I can hear, I can hear pretty well, except I still have problems in restaurants. People who can hear tell me they have the same problem.

Richard: Normal people hearing have- Janet Fox: Right, right.

Richard: Problems at restaurants.

Janet Fox: But I think it's more exaggerated for me because I hear everything all at once. I'm learning to filter. And hear things differently. It's a process, the whole thing is a process. But I was wearing a hearing aid in my right ear, a ReSound, which works with the Cochlear. And it's kind of balanced things out in the beginning, but at this point it's not working anymore.

COCHLEARIMPLANTBASICS.COM

Richard: You're having a progressive loss in your hearing aid ear?

Janet Fox: Right. It just makes things very shrill.

Richard: There's less comprehension in your hearing aid ear now and that's what's causing the problem. You've considered getting a second implant for that ear, right?

Janet Fox: Right.

Richard: Three years later is a long time for a lot of people. I'd like to know what's going through your mind right now. About the second one?

Janet Fox: Well, I notice myself leaning in with my left ear to hear everybody because I can't hear anything in this ear. And it's just like before. I'm getting half of everything.

Richard: Does your brother have two cochlear?

Janet Fox: No.

Richard: He has one.

Janet Fox: He has one.

Richard: And he's getting along?

Janet Fox: He says he is. I can see the difference though. He is better. He is much better. But he still has that blank look a lot. You know which look I'm talking about.

Richard: Yes I do.

Janet Fox: He's supportive of me. He wouldn't do it though. He has issues too because his wife has Alzheimer's. He has like 10% hearing, and you don't want to lose that.

Richard: That's not uncommon, because some people I've known had 4% in one ear and afraid to lose it. But you're not in that position anymore. You want to move forward.

Janet Fox: Well, you know I have like 10 or 20% in this ear yet, so I can hear noise. I can hear stuff like that. But in the big picture, I can't hear. I'm really not losing anything.

Richard: You said to me before, you were nervous about the second operation. And I'm sure people who are listening to this podcast would like to know how you're feeling about going back in for surgery for a second cochlear implant.

Janet Fox: Well, the thoughts that keep going through my head, is it could be twice as good or twice as bad. I'm going to hear things in stereo. What I'm looking forward to is being able to adjust my own volume and everything on my phone. This is a biggie for me. I'm tired of carrying around all those gadgets. I'm excited. I am.

Richard: And nervous at the same time?

Janet Fox: Yeah. It's like going on a trip. You know, some place you've never been before.

Richard: Fear makes us move forward.

Janet Fox: Right. Yeah. You either move forward or you go back. And I'm not going back.

Richard: No.

Janet Fox: No. I can't go back.

Richard: Right now, you're using the Cochlear Nucleus 6.

Janet Fox: Yeah.

Richard: And when you get implanted on the other side, you'll be able to upgrade to 7 for both sides.

Janet Fox: I'll have two 7's.

Richard: Two 7's. Excellent. Okay.

Janet Fox: I'll have two 7's and a 6 on the side.

Richard: As a backup.

Janet Fox: The backup, yeah.

Richard: Sure. You've never used the Kanso? You've never used one, have you?

Janet Fox: No.

Richard: No. Okay.

Janet Fox: Have you? Richard: I have both. So- Janet Fox: You like it?

Richard: I use it for different purposes. I don't use it that much. I agree. The 7 is much better. Okay.

Janet Fox: Yeah, okay.

Richard: And so somewhere down the road you're hoping for the stereo sound, better comprehension. Fine. Okay. And I hope in a couple of months from now after you've been activated, you're going to sit down with me and talk about what it's like after surgery. Because I know a lot of listeners would like to know your experience. There are lots of people sitting on the fence. Do you have anything you would tell people sitting on the fence that can be helpful to them?

Janet Fox: Jump.

Richard: All right.

Janet Fox: Really. I mean, at the point when I realized how bad my hearing was, it was like I said, the more forward you go back, and I'm not going back. You know?

Janet Fox: I'm never going to regain my hearing. I will never hear like I used to hear. So, I have to learn how to hear differently. It's an adventure. It can be frustrating. But I would take this over being deaf any day. I can hear. Sometimes I walk around in the morning without the cochlear on just to have the quiet. But I find myself missing it because I like hearing. I like hearing noise; I like hearing my dog. I like hearing ... Well music I need to work a lot on. That's one thing I do miss.

Richard: Did you enjoy music before?

Janet Fox: I love music. Well, yeah, I think that helped with the hearing loss. I went to a lot of concerts, a lot. You know, we're coming from the 50s, 60s, and 70s, a lot of rock and roll.

Richard: You know you can get that back? Yes you can.

Janet Fox: Well, I'm going to work on it.

Richard: Good. All right.

Janet Fox: I am.

Janet Fox: But that's the only thing that I'm missing right now. I can have conversations with people. I'm having a conversation with you. I couldn't have a conversation before. And now I'm looking forward to having one in stereo.

Richard: And having one in groups.

Janet Fox: Oh, groups.

Richard: You'll be able to do.

Janet Fox: Yeah, this is one of the things-

Richard: What's going on with when you have a conversation with a group? What happens?

Janet Fox: This is one of the deciding factors of getting a second one. We went out to dinner with some friends, and I was sitting in the middle of two women, and I could only hear the conversation on my left. I couldn't hear the conversation; I couldn't hear the woman's sitting next to me.

Richard: And you constantly have to turn your head?

Janet Fox: Right.

Richard: Your head will fall off with time.

Janet Fox: I'm going to unscrew myself here.

Janet Fox: So, I was like, "This is crazy." When I got tested for the second one, they said, "You're definitely a candidate. No problem."

Richard: All right, so what we'll do is in two months from now, we'll sit down again, and we'll see what your progress is. Good, bad, or indifferent. Because what I'm trying to do with my podcasts is present an unvarnished truth. I want people to know without the influence of a manufacturer involved, that this is what people are actually experiencing. It's very helpful.

Janet Fox: Oh yeah. We just came back from a steamboat cruise down the Mississippi. It was lovely. And I was standing there one day, I don't know where we were on the ship, but this woman comes over to me, taps me on the back and points to her head. You know?

Janet Fox: And she had a cochlear too. Along the trip we would bump into each other and there was a lot of people. We talked about, "Can you hear them? Do you understand what they're saying?" You know, some of it, a lot of it in large crowds we had the same thing. But she was also thinking about getting a second one. We had a lot of common.

Richard: Excellent. That's very, very good. Very interesting.

Janet Fox: Yeah.

Richard: You may motivate people to move ahead.

Janet Fox: I hope so. I do. I really do. Jump. Really,

Richard: That's what I tell people. If it doesn't work out, you can always take the processor off your head. You're no worse off than you are.

Janet Fox: And I'll be exactly where I was before I couldn't hear. It's funny because I've been wearing this for three years and I know some people think I can hear like normal people because we have conversations like normal people. And I forget until I take it off. Then everything is like ... But I also have tinnitus, so I never have a silent moment.

Richard: Well, let's talk about that. That's very, very interesting. How bad is it on a one to 10 scale?

Janet Fox: Nine.

Janet Fox: Yeah. I've had a long time, a long, long time. Some say it's an indication that you have a hearing problem. I've had this at least 25 years.

Richard: And sometimes, often actually, a cochlear implant will reduce the amount of tinnitus. Let's hope in two months from now you can tell me how it's working out.

Janet Fox: The tinnitus gets worse under stress. Okay?

Richard: True.

Janet Fox: Without the cochlear on, if I'm stressed, it's really loud. If I'm not too stressed, it's not too bad. With the cochlear on, it's not bad at all.

Richard: It is reducing?

Janet Fox: Yeah, it helps. It really helps.

Richard: So hopefully with the second one it will help even more.

Janet Fox: I'm sure it will. It's like now I'm not wearing my hearing aid and I have the tinnitus. I can hear it on this side.

Richard: It doesn't go throughout your whole head it's one side or the other?

Janet Fox: Well, it does, but when I don't have something to distract, I can hear it more.

Richard: Okay.

Janet Fox: It's very annoying.

Richard: I'm sure it must be. I'm sure it must be. All right. What we'll do is we'll plan to talk again in a couple of months. And of course, I wish you all the best. I'm sure Dr. Wazen one of the finest surgeons in the area, and he'll do his best for you.

Janet Fox: I'll tell you; he did beautiful work. Beautiful.

Richard: Excellent. Okay, Janet. Thank you so much for your time.

Janet Fox: You're welcome.

CHAPTER 10 JANET FOX PART 2

THE DIFFERENCES THAT BILATERAL HEARING MAKES

Janet Fox recently received a second cochlear implant and became a bilateral recipient. This is Part 2, the follow up interview done after her second cochlear implant activation.

Part 1 of her interview was done just prior to her operation. At the time we sat down for that interview it was my stated intention to do another after she was activated with the new one.

Many cochlear implant recipients who are qualified for a second one hesitate for a variety of reasons; fear of losing any residual hearing in their other ear; loss of fidelity of music if they still have any residual hearing and sometimes being in denial, believing and stating that one ear is good enough to get by with.

Janet moved beyond that point, realizing that after more than two years after receiving her first cochlear implant that her remaining hearing was in decline and of no practical use. It was time to take the plunge.

Drs. Wazen and Nayak at Silverstein Institute in Sarasota, who performed her original surgery also did the second. They complied with an unusual request from Janet which she talks about.

Although her activation was very recent, she already sees the results and the improvement. I felt it was time for her to share experience while it is still new. I was also interested in her reaction to her upgrades from having a single side Cochlear Nucleus 6 to becoming a bilateral Nucleus 7 recipient.

She wrote to me in a follow up communication after the interview:

"BTW you can quote me saying, I'll never take this off, and it's so great to hear in stereo!"

Richard: I interviewed Janet Fox just prior to her recent surgery where she had a second cochlear implant operation. My stated objective was to capture her experiences on both sides of being bimodal with a hearing aid on one side, and post operation of now being bilateral with cochlear implants on both. Originally I intended to wait a few months post op and post activation to let her hearing normalize. Upon reflection, I decided to move that interview forward in order to capture her experience without the passage of time and forgetfulness. In other words, to express her feelings and record her experiences while undergoing the fine tuning or the mapping of her new processors. We discuss the differences between her first operation and the second, the results, and her expectations for the future. In our post interview communication she wrote, "By the way, you can quote me saying I'll never take this off. It's so great to hear in stereo."

Richard: We recently did an interview and you were preparing to have the second side operated on to receive bilateral cochlear implant.

Janet Fox: Correct.

Richard: What made you decide to go ahead and get the second one?

Janet Fox: What made me decide?

Richard: Yeah.

Janet Fox: I couldn't hear out of my right ear. It was just deteriorating more and more, so I found myself leaning in with my left ear to hear people, and if somebody sat to my right, I couldn't hear them. I can only hear the people on my left. I think that was a good indication I needed something more.

Richard: Okay. And how many weeks ago did you have the second one done?

Janet Fox: Four. I have done October 1st.

Richard: Oh, exactly four weeks.

Janet Fox: Yeah.

Richard: Okay. And Dr. Wazen was the surgeon this time?

Janet Fox: Correct. He was the surgeon last time too.

Richard: Okay.

Janet Fox: And Dr. Nayak. They did a beautiful job in the surgery. They really did.

Richard: What were the differences in your mind about getting the first one done and the second one done regarding surgery? Were you more afraid, less afraid?

Janet Fox: I wasn't afraid, but I'm very vain. I am. I said to him before the surgery, "Listen, I have very short hair, so you have to make sure they're even in the back." And they did. They measured everything. They did a beautiful job. I wasn't anxious about the surgery itself. I know Dr. Wazen is good because he did the other one. He did a good job. So no, I wasn't concerned about it. And just going through the surgery, it was a process. Waking up from the surgery this time was different.

Richard: What was different about it?

Janet Fox: It was horrible. Last time I didn't have any repercussions from the anesthesia and this time I did. And the pain in my head, I felt got hit by a Mack Truck. It was bad.

Richard: Did they have any idea why it was different the second time? They never discussed it with you?

Janet Fox: No. They don't know why, but I need to find out the name of the anesthesia, so I don't get it again because I had a bad reaction to it.

Richard: Then somebody going in for surgery, they should know what the anesthesia is, discuss it and if they've had surgery before to discuss that with the anesthesiologist.

Janet Fox: Yeah. As far as I know it was the same. Now I don't know how much my diet has to do with it because I'm eating very clean, so everything affects me.

Richard: That makes sense. All right. And then so the postop was different? You just felt sicker?

Janet Fox: Yeah, I was sick for like two days. It was not good. And then I came home, and I just slept.

Richard: Which is probably a good thing to do.

Janet Fox: Feeling like that, yeah. The first one, I didn't have any of that. And the first one I just remember just going home and sleeping, and then being okay, but not with this one.

Richard: Was this one vertigo or was it pain?

Janet Fox: No, I had vertigo. I opened my eyes and the whole turned sideways once. Yeah, it happened once. I thought I was falling out of bed. Thank God it only happened once.

Richard: And what about the pain? Was there a lot of pain this time?

Janet Fox: Yeah, there was a lot of pain.

Richard: What did you take?

Janet Fox: Well, they gave me a very, very strong painkiller narcotic, which didn't agree with me either. I had to stop taking that and I just started taking Tylenol.

Richard: Okay. And then you had to wait how many weeks until you are activated on this one?

Janet Fox: Three.

Richard: Three weeks you waited?

Janet Fox: Yeah. It was three weeks, and the activation was very different. This whole thing is very different than the first one.

Richard: Let's talk about that for a bit. What was different?

Janet Fox: When I got the first one activated, I could understand voices. I could distinguish what they were saying. With this one, everything is just garbled. There's no understanding. It's just a lot of noise when I'm wearing just the one. The new one.

Richard: The new one.

Janet Fox: Yeah.

Richard: But it's only been how many weeks now?

Janet Fox: Three weeks.

Richard: It'll be three weeks.

Janet Fox: But I want miracles.

Richard: Two weeks. So right now, you're still relatively new with the new side and it's not clear enough yet. It should get better with time.

Janet Fox: It's not clear on itself. Paired with the first cochlear I can hear very well. I went out to lunch with three other women in a noisy restaurant and I heard say 90% of the conversation.

Janet Fox: Yeah. That's what I said. I could actually hear people.

Richard: It's been years since you did that.

Janet Fox: Yeah, it's been a long time. On itself, I can't ... Well, I just had an adjustment today, so I don't know what's going to happen when I take the other one off. I have no idea yet. As far as feeling goes, I'm feeling very vulnerable since the surgery.

Richard: You want to describe that a bit? Vulnerable how?

Janet Fox: Just kind of shaky. It's like I'm not sure what's going to happen.

Richard: With your hearing?

Janet Fox: Well yeah, and my emotional wellbeing. It's a scary experience. You hope for the best and then you hear tin. Then I remember what happened with the first one. I heard better but it was still tinny, but it improved over time and practice. I got to practice too.

Richard: The new one, it's tinny now, but hopefully as you practice more it will clear up and then you should be able to use either one independently if you had to, but right now, no.

Janet Fox: Well yeah, I can use the left one independently. Already, in such a short period of time, found that I've been dependent on the right one because I hear so much better with two.

Richard: Two ears are better than one.

Janet Fox: Oh, they are. That's why God gave us two.

Richard: That's true. The fine tuning this morning was your second. Today was your second mapping with the fine tuning and they basically did what today?

Janet Fox: They basically raised the volume.

Richard: They haven't added any SCAN programs to it yet?

Janet Fox: No, nothing yet. Nothing.

Richard: Which is not unusual. Usually, the first three or four they just keep getting your brain used to the volume and then they worry about the SCANs later.

Janet Fox: Yeah, that's what he told me. He said, "Don't worry about anything, but just get the volume. And then after we're on the fifth one, we'll start working with playing around with everything."

Richard: Excellent. That's good. You don't regret having the second one.

Janet Fox: Oh no. No, I don't. I mean I could have told myself, and my brother does this, I had that 10% hearing, that's good enough. It's not. I still have a little residual hearing.

Richard: I was about to ask you about that. Tell me about what you feel with the residual hearing.

Janet Fox: I can hear things drop, loud noise. I can't hear my dog bark, but I can hear loud noises. I feel things more than hear them, I think. I was surprised I could hear anything at all.

Richard: That's one thing that a lot of people are afraid of is losing any residual hearing, but the understanding I have is that the surgical techniques have improved so much that retaining residual hearing is becoming more common. Did the surgeon discuss that with you?

Janet Fox: No.

Richard: Not really. Okay.

Janet Fox: No. I think he may have discussed it the first time I had it.

But the residual hearing that's there is minimal.

Richard: Does it give you any confidence you have any left at all?

Janet Fox: No.

Richard: No. Okay. That's fine. That's a good point. And your advice to somebody who is thinking about getting the second one, sitting on the fence saying that my bad ear is good enough. Do you have any advice for them?

Janet Fox: Well, pay real close attention to the ear that you don't have the cochlear on, and really be honest with yourself in self-evaluation of how you're hearing. Like I was saying, my brother does the same thing, and he says, "Well, it's good enough." When push comes to shove, it wasn't good enough for me.

Richard: You know that's a very interesting point you said to me before because your brother has the single side cochlear implant. He was using you as a guinea pig to see what the second side is like.

Janet Fox: Probably. Well now he's going to get all my tools. I had the N6, now I had the N7, which is really a nice upgrade. I can talk on the phone without having the phone clip, which I love. I don't need all that stuff; I'm giving it all to my brother. He still has the N6.

Richard: That's Great. Well, what do you have for backup? If this fails, you keep one? You keep the processor though.

Janet Fox: I have an N6, yeah. I'm keeping that, but I have multiple tools that I won't use.

Richard: Excellent, so maybe your brother will listen. Now, let me ask you another question. The differences between the N6 and the N7, because people often say, "Should I bother upgrade?" Is it worth it?

Janet Fox: Yeah, I mean just to have access to the phone, like the phone rings, I can pick it up. I think the sound is better.

Richard: I found the sound to be more robust. Do you find it clearer?
Janet Fox: It's mellower, I would say.

Janet Fox: Yeah. That the N6, but again, I'm still getting used to it, but I like it better. I do.

Richard: I wanted to sit down and talk to you so soon after you were activated with the second side because I wanted to be sure your memory was fresh.

Janet Fox: Oh, it's fresh.

Richard: Okay, that's good. Do you have anything you'd like to add to people who are sitting on the fence?

Janet Fox: I would say go for it. I just say go for it.

Richard: Okay, that's great.

Janet Fox: Like the first one, go for it.

Richard: That's great. Okay Janet, I thank you so much for your time and I'm sure that people are going to be interested in listening to part two of our interview. If you're thinking about going bilateral you can take some of Janet's experience and use that to make your decision. Thank you so much.

Janet Fox: Thank you.

CHAPTER 11 JACK BARNES

A PEDIATRIC COCHLEAR IMPLANT RECIPIENT THIRTY-THREE YEARS LATER

Jack Barnes was implanted in 1988 when he was 11 after suffering a total sudden hearing loss. It was an experimental process at the time.

Thirty-three years later is still using the original surgical implant but is now on the 8th generation of external, improved technology. He recently received a Cochlear Nucleus 7. He is a unique resource who has traveled the entire road of the history of cochlear implants. Inspirational because of his perseverance and, as you will discover, his unstoppable drive in his endeavors.

Richard: Jack Barnes is one of those unforgettable characters I've met along my hearing journey. I had received my bilateral cochlear implant surgery about a year before I met him. I had treated my processors with extreme caution, afraid to damage them and lose my precious gift of hearing. Then I attended a presentation that Jack gave with a slideshow. He was running marathons in the pouring rain while wearing his external Cochlear processor. Cochlear tough was the only descriptive term I could think of. There was no sport, aside from boxing, which was restricted by wearing a cochlear implant.

Jack was implanted in 1988 when he was 11 after suffering a total sudden hearing loss. There was an experimental process at the time. He is still using the original surgical implant but is now on the eighth generation of external improved technology. Cochlear is always backwards compatible.

Jack Barnes: Absolutely. It's good to speak with you, sir. This is Jack Barnes. It's Tuesday, February 16th, 2021, and we're speaking from Miami, Florida.

Richard: Excellent. Tell me a little bit about your hearing loss. How did it happen?

Jack Barnes: This goes all the way back to 1987. I was a normal hearing child with no problems at all, and quite suddenly, contracted meningitis, which turned out to be bacterial and presented very much like the flu. I went from very nearly perfect hearing to no hearing overnight, very abrupt. And just happened to be by way of luck and circumstance, the cochlear implant had recently become available as an experimental surgery for children. And I was fortunate to receive the implant about a year later in 1988.

Richard: How old were you then?

Jack Barnes: I was about 11 going to 12 at that point. I've now had the same internal Nucleus 22 cochlear implant for over 33 years.

Richard: And you've never had a problem with it?

Jack Barnes: Not a single day has it been anything other than completely reliable.

Richard: I remember when I first started investigating cochlear implants, that Cochlear said that the internal should last about 73 years. My re-implantation surgery, the surgeon hasn't been born yet.

Jack Barnes: You've already got it on the calendar, I noticed. In my case, when the implant was discussed, it was brand new. It's never been done before. There wasn't any kind of concrete guidance as to how long it might last within in the internal implant. I've been extremely fortunate that the initial guidance that was provided has long since been exceeded, and I'm now on my eighth platform for external sound processors.

Richard: Explain what the platform is about. People-

Jack Barnes: Sure thing. There are two components of the device that together create sound for me, one being the internal implant, which is what is physically embedded into the inner ear cochlea. And then the external processor, which engages by way of magnetic connection and passes the programming to the internal implant. The external sound processor also has the microphones that capture sound and pass through the coding to render the sound processing on the inside. The eighth generation that I'm using now was the Nucleus 7 for the N22 internal.

Richard: Which was the first one you used?

Jack Barnes: I began with the WSP, the Wearable Speech Processor, and this had three AA batteries. And you will remember the Sony Walkman. It was about the size of a Sony Walkman with three AAA's that I would wear in a hip pack on my waist.

Richard: The funny thing is that you're now mentioned you're on the eighth and you've had it for 33 years. We are talking about an upgrade approximately every four years.

Jack Barnes: About every four years. That's where I am on average, which is really incredible when you think about it. Right now, you and I are speaking utilizing technologies, one of them being Bluetooth, which didn't exist when I received my internal implant. The way in which the manufacturers, in my case, Cochlear, has made a choice to continue making the new external processor backwards compatible with Legacy internal implants, advancing the technology, and incorporating it in the external sound processor is amazing.

Richard: I need to ask you about the N22 implant. There was an issue for a long time about getting the Nucleus 7 compatible with it. Can you give us a little background or why that was?

Jack Barnes: I can't speak to the company side of that. I can only say that certainly the Nucleus 6, which I participated in the launch, which was definitely on the market. I want to say this goes back to 2015. From that average we were just discussing that period from N6 to N7 was about as expected from my view.

Richard: Okay, but you had an issue. The N22 was not compatible with the N7 for several years, two or three years.

Jack Barnes: Yes. The Nucleus 7 launched in 2017 and it was originally compatible within the N24 implant. As is always the case, the manufacturers wanted to serve and showcase the current offering with the broadest possible number of users. In the case of myself and other pioneers of the technology, there aren't all that many of us left, and so it's a great testament to the company itself that they choose to make that device backward compatible at all. But it's a very strong expectation of mine that many of the things that are on the internal modern implants, that the external device relies upon to communicate, don't exist in my internal implant.

Jack Barnes: I would imagine there were very significant technological and engineering challenges that had to be overcome to create an N7 that's compatible with my device. It's my experience that each cycle of update for the external processors, there's usually at least a year lag, sometimes more, between when the processor first comes to market and when it's offered for Legacy users. In this case, the duration of time from when the Nucleus 7 was offered for the N22 was not out of line at all with my expectations.

Very happy to receive it.

Richard: Now I want to go back a step. You were about 11 when you had the implant. Tell me about how your parents reacted to it when you lost your hearing.

Jack Barnes: I would imagine they weren't happy about that. Probably not the most pleasant of moments for anyone. But we were certainly excited about the prospect of the cochlear implant, which they had no knowledge of before I lost my hearing. But it just turned out that we were living in Phoenix at the time, and one of the centers in America that was at the forefront of implant technology as well as process, was the House Ear Institute in Los Angeles, which was close enough that we were able to make direct and frequent visits to House Ear. And it turned out that not only was I a candidate, but they had strong optimism about the outcomes that I might receive. Both of my parents were enthusiastically in support of the process.

Jack Barnes: One thing that not everyone knows about cochlear implantation is that once you've lost your hearing entirely, as I like to say, there's no downside. If it completely fails, I'm going to be exactly as I was before I got the implant. And certainly, in my case, the outcomes were and had been extraordinary. The prospect of my remaining hearing was definitely a very strong positive for my parents. And they were in the support of my receiving the device.

Richard: Did they do two at the same time? Was it bilateral surgery?

Jack Barnes: Back in the day, there really wasn't bilateral implantation. Certainly not as prominent as it is today. As an experimental surgery, when I received the cochlear implant, the focus was proving that it worked at all for children, and it was not until I would say at least 20 years after I received the device, that bilateral implantation became as common practice as it is today.

Richard: Do you have two now or just one?

Jack Barnes: I only have the one now.

Richard: Have you ever considered going for the second?

Jack Barnes: I have, and I've had several consultations with surgeons, and they assure me that while it can be done, the quality of sound is unknown, given that so many years have passed in the time that I have not heard out of the unimplanted ear. I know that you yourself probably have views on how that works.

Richard: I was totally deaf for 35 years and the sound is perfectly natural. So again, yes, it can be a crapshoot, but the length of deafness is not necessarily an indicator that it won't work.

Jack Barnes: Nope. And no one has suggested it wouldn't.

Richard: You get the cochlear implant. You're now in junior high school.

Jack Barnes: Just before. It was at the end of elementary school going into junior high.

Richard: How did you do in school with the cochlear implant?

Jack Barnes: I was very lucky in my teachers, when I lost my hearing, were very supportive and I remained in the mainstream classroom. I spent the remainder of a full academic year without being able to hear at all and benefited from sympathetic teachers, lip-reading teacher, who was a speech language pathologist who helped me develop some skill and understanding without being able to hear. And very sympathetic classroom students who took notes in some cases on my behalf. I was very grateful for support all around.

Jack Barnes: Once I received the implant, the following summer was the start of sixth grade that I entered with the benefit of the cochlear implant. And it helped tremendously. And then it really became the foundation for all the success that was [inaudible 00:12:41].

152

Richard: How'd you deal with the telephone with one ear?

Jack Barnes: With the telephone it was a challenge. I used the TDD for a while. As a matter of fact, that was the thing back in the late 80s. The TDD was very helpful for me, as I relearned to hear using the device with the phone. Over time, which became very natural for me as well. The first job that I received coming out of college was in commercial finance, making telephone calls all day long. The acceleration and the adoption period was pretty rapid. It worked out very well.

Richard: In college, you didn't have a problem because of your hearing?

Jack Barnes: Only in very select cases. I happened to have one economics professor who was the co-author of a principle that had won the Nobel Prize in Economics, who just so happened to have the deepest voice and the least expressive face in the history of spoken language. I did reach out and see if we can get some assistance in better understanding that specific individual. But for the most part, the classroom setting has been one that's always been very comfortable for me. I sit up at the front of the class and I'm engaging and connect directly with professors to better understand what I can do to capture more of the lesson. Worked out very well.

Richard: I must tell the story here that I first met you at a Cochlear convention and you were the speaker. And I had been implanted just over a year before, and I was treating my cochlear implants like they were delicate instruments. You stood up on the stage with your slideshow of running marathons in the rain with a cochlear implant.

Jack Barnes: That's true.

Richard: Suddenly it turned my entire perspective around. Let's talk a little bit about what IP ratings are, the waterproof aspect of the cochlear implant, and how they affected you.

Jack Barnes: So, IP V6, IP V7, these are different standards, different ratings that define both the depth and duration that devices generally can be submerged in water. I can assure you that I have pressed well beyond the limits of all of these ratings both intentionally and unintentionally across my devices, and the most recent cochlear device has been extraordinary. The Nucleus 6, Nucleus 7 are amazing in their water resistance. As a Floridian yourself, you'll know that we do not lack for opportunity to test things out in water, and both swimming as well as in the rain walking my dogs, it's a tremendous re-insurance that I can be outside with these most modern devices and not have concern that the devices will suffer for humidity or direct water exposure.

Jack Barnes: I was in Fiji traveling early 2000s, alone, rolling through the Colo-i-Suva Forest, crossing a creek. And I dropped my then implant, which I think was the 3G, but don't quote me on that. One of the earlier devices. And I dropped it right into the river and pulled it out and panicked, dried it off, and fortunately was able to regain some functionality as we went. But the degree of confidence that we have in these most modern devices is amazing in terms of their waterproofness and environmental toughness.

Richard: Talk to me about music. How do you deal with music?

Jack Barnes: Cannot more strongly recommend music as a training technique for relearning to hear. I'm often misunderstood when I use this word training practice. People think I'm talking about hard work. I guess, to a certain degree, I am. But everything is training. Everything is practice. This conversation, it's training and practice. And it's that intentional, purposeful listening that I think creates the breakthroughs that help us understand spoken words in context. And [inaudible 00:16:48] to distinguish hearing from understanding. For me, listening to music has been one of the most important tools for enjoyment, but even beyond enjoyment, learning to understand spoken words [inaudible 00:17:04].

Jack Barnes: One of the things that I'm wanting to do when I lost my hearing and then regained it with the Nucleus 22, was better understand how I could understand what people were saying in noisy environments, which was not easy for me at the time. I bought a copy of the Beastie Boys Licensed to Ill and opened the inner jacket, the liner with all the lyrics on the inside. And I played it at intolerable decibels, as often as I could, reading the words, as I listened to the songs. And over time it became a very strong tool for distinguishing spoken words in the midst of background noise.

Jack Barnes: Beyond the joy that is listening to music, I think it's an also important opportunity for those with hearing impairment, and certainly those with cochlear implants to train and to listen with intention.

Richard: It's interesting you should say that because one of the rehabilitation techniques I recommend to people are YouTube music videos, but you must also put in the word, with lyrics, because the brain needs the lyrics to start to make sense of everything. And it works. It's a great technique. Music is a great trainer. You've traveled. Nothing to stop you.

Jack Barnes: Travel is a joy. Travel is just a joy. Unfortunately, the year 2020 did put a significant crimp in our travel plans, as it did for most others who enjoy like we do, but we're very, very much looking forward to it. One of the more recent trips that we took, my wife and I, was just under a month that we did in China. And we originally started where we had been a MakeA-Wish Southern Florida gala that had a pre-gala auction. And we purchased a weekend in Shanghai.

Jack Barnes: And somehow a weekend in Shanghai became a 28-day trip across China that included a week's long study of Kung Fu at the Shaolin Temple in Dongfeng. We tested the ability of the Nucleus 6 to withstand sweat and humidity in Dongfeng. But travel is an incredible opportunity, and I cannot more encourage travel generally, but certainly for those with implants, because it presents such an opportunity to consume new experience.

Richard: On the other side of that page, I traveled for 35 years with no hearing, including the circumnavigation of the world. And I could never hear the tour guides and I had to buy books of every port we were going to and read up before I got there. I'm looking forward one day to doing travel again with hearing. It makes a big, big difference.

Richard: Let me ask you another question here about what would you like to see in the future of the next generation of cochlear implant, the processor?

Jack Barnes: From an internal perspective, well, internal external hearing [inaudible 00:20:14], one of the things that excites me are the increasing duration with which power will last. The Nucleus 7 that I've just received has the benefit of batteries that are powered by USB connection, which means that I now have much less concern about being able to hear if there's ever a hurricane that knocks out power, because I have battery packs and generators that can now power the batteries. But the degree of independence, I think, that will result from either longer-powered devices or maybe even fully implanted device are both very, very exciting. I think there are some technological hurdles by way the skin flap and how waterproofing works with microphones before we get all the way to fully implanted devices. But it's hard to think that that's not on the radar at some point.

Richard: That's a very interesting point because the new Nucleus Kanso 2 is rechargeable only. And now I'm watching on social media, people in Kansas and Texas with no power for two or three days, they can't charge them up. It's still the battery issue. Yes, I agree that the batteries have gotten better, especially something called the Vartas, V-A-R-T-A-S battery, which has been able to increase the power of the lithium side. The future for battery power is absolutely astounding.

Richard: What else would you like to add to this? Would you like to tell people who were thinking about getting a cochlear implant you've walked in their moccasins? What would you tell them?

Jack Barnes: I would tell them not to wait. Time is short. Time is the one resource that is truly scarce. And each day that we go without hearing, or at least each day that we go without hearing for fear of what the process to regaining hearing might be like, is a day that separates us from the possibilities of life. And that's a concern to me that there might be people avoiding this conversation or avoiding signing up for the clinical examinations that might lead on the path to cochlear implantation. I would say don't hesitate. There is no downside. Certainly, there are considerations. Certainly, there are implications, but I would not want for anyone considering this process, this technology, this opportunity, from a lens of fear, there's just no reason to.

Richard:

That's absolutely on point. Jack, I wanted to thank you for taking your time. I'm sure you're going to be helping many, many people with this interview. Thank you very much.

Jack Barnes:

Thank you for having me.

CHAPTER 12 KATHY COMBS

EITHER THE TESTING MACHINERY IS BROKEN OR MY HEARING IS

Kathy discovered her hearing loss while self-testing an audiometer as a school nurse. She realized that either the machine had a problem or her hearing. It was her hearing.

Many will be able to relate to her succession of unfulfilling hearing aid solutions. She adapted to a series of vocational changes within the nursing field. Kathy struggled every step of the way.

That is, until eventually, she found the right help and received a cochlear implant. Today she has a Cochlear Nucleus 6 on side and an Oticon Agile Pro hearing aid on the other and is considering a second implant. In the interim, she is constantly discovering new situations where she can function at a high level with better hearing.

Richard: My guest today is Kathy Combs. Kathy has a long, varied career in the nursing field, and she discovered her hearing loss while selftesting an audiometer while working as a school nurse. She realized either the machine was broken or her hearing. It turned out to be her hearing. She talks about her series of missteps along the way. There are expensive hearing aids that did not provide improved speech comprehension for her, but luxury vacations for the hearing aid dealer. She eventually qualified for a cochlear implant, and it changed her life. Today she has a Cochlear Nucleus 6 on one side, and a hearing aid on the other. And she talks about why she is considering a cochlear implant for the other side.

NOTE: Kathy Combs received her second implant in 2021 and is now bilateral.

Kathy Combs: My hearing loss probably started before I became aware of it. I used to be a school nurse in Massachusetts in the 90s into the 2000s and part of my job was doing hearing screening on the students. And so, of course, I would test the equipment prior to using it on myself. And I realized either the equipment was faulty, or it was my hearing that was faulty. I also had discovered I was having difficulty speaking with several people.

Richard: How long ago was that?

Kathy Combs: That was back in, probably in my forties. So, I decided to get it evaluated. I did go to my primary care, who I believe wasn't doing hearing screenings at that time or referred me to an ENT. So, I went to an ENT who had an audiologist in his office, and she diagnosed bilateral hearing loss. She also suggested hearing aids, but at that time she was not quote, "Selling or prescribing or offering hearing aids out of her office."

Kathy Combs: And so, with minimal guidance, I went to look for a place that sold hearing aids. I probably did the worst thing you could have done without guidance; I went to a place that was in a mall where I should've had some suspicion that the person, who was a salesperson, not an audiologist, I came to realize, was telling me about trips that he got to take. Well, those trips were probably based on the amount of hearing aids he sold, so I fell for it. I bought one. He recommended two, but at the time I thought I will just try the one. And I believe at that time was my left ear where I bought the one hearing aid.

Richard: Did it help you at all?

Kathy Combs: It did help me; it did help me. And so-

Richard: How about with your job? You were working as a nurse. Were you able to communicate? Was it clear?

Kathy Combs: Yes, yes, it did help. So that was fine for a while, but it wasn't perfect, and I kept going back, ultimately... Trying to think, a couple of years went by, and I did go to somebody else who recommended Widex hearing aids. So, those were my first bilateral hearing aids, and they were very good, they were very helpful. But then I felt like I was fine with the job and with these new hearing aids. And so that probably went on for another five more years, but then again, I found they weren't doing quite as well as I had hoped.

Richard: You're deteriorating as your hearing was deteriorating [crosstalk 00:00:05:25].

Kathy Combs: Exactly.

Richard: And you were still doing your job at the time?

Kathy Combs: I was still doing my job, but I felt sometimes, because I was working with school-aged children, and their voices are higher frequencies that I really was noticing more difficulty hearing the kids. As it turned out in 2008, my husband, his position in Massachusetts transferred here to Florida. So, I left the job, I retired and came here, and considered at that time perhaps still pursuing school nursing, which I really loved, and I had done probably a total of 15 years in Massachusetts.

Kathy Combs: However, the school system is a little different here. Instead of one nurse in every school, there's an LPN in most of the schools and the RN supervises one, or more, schools. So, for me, realizing that I did have a hearing loss, that it was all new kids, all new schools, all new staff, it dawned on me that this is probably not the best option for me work-wise. So, I did what I had also done part-time in Massachusetts, I went into home

160

care, so private duty home care. And that wasn't too much of a struggle because I'd be one-on-one, or one-on-one, with the patient, the client and the family. And again, not too difficult.

Kathy Combs: My hearing did not improve, continued to decrease. I came to a new audiologist here in Florida, probably two years after I moved here. And she recommended upgrading my hearing aids because the technology, et cetera, et cetera. One thing that I always find interesting is, when I was in Massachusetts, the hearing aid provider there told me about telecoils. So, I had great Widex hearing aids with telecoils that I never used because there really wasn't much looped, or I didn't know much about looping. I came to Florida and my new audiologist talks about, "Do you want a telecoil?" And I thought, "Well, I didn't really use it too much when I was in Massachusetts, what do you think?"

Kathy Combs: And she said, "Well, it will make the hearing aid a little heavier." What I wish she had told me is, "You're in Florida now, there are dozens of venues that are looped." There are churches, houses of worship, there are so many places that are looped. "Yes, I think it's a great idea here." She didn't tell me that. So, I ended up with my new hearing aids, which were Oticon's, and ultimately had to get a streamer for those because they didn't have the little nifty telecoil adapter.

Kathy Combs: Anyhow, that did seem to work for a while. I would go back periodically, I think every year, for a reevaluation and my hearing did not improve. So, it continued to regress.

Richard: Did you find yourself getting more isolated?

Kathy Combs: I did and it's sad. People talk about isolation. I think with that isolation, somebody might've mentioned today, just that sadness that you can't communicate with people anymore. That is so much of a challenge.

Kathy Combs: In fact, I just remember being anxious before going into the booth because I pretty much knew that it wasn't better, that it was worse. And she finally said, "I haven't done this too many times, but I really think you might need to see somebody else."

Kathy Combs: So initially, I believe she referred me to a doctor, an ENT, who suggested an MRI to see if there was anything new, different, that might have affected the hearing, and there wasn't. At that point she said, "I think you should think about a cochlear implant as an option." Richard: Did you know about them?

Kathy Combs: I knew about them. I think at that point I had been in Florida a couple of years, maybe it was later than that, Richard. Maybe it was 2012. I can't remember because I didn't follow through right away on that suggestion. I had gone to a few HLAA meetings, but became much more active in the group after... Do you remember Joan Haber? So, Joan became a mentor, I would say to me, in terms of helping me just talk about what an implant involves.

Richard: I'm curious, what was your feeling about implants that time? You've been told now you might qualify for one, or you qualify for one. Do you remember what you felt at the time? Were you afraid?

Kathy Combs: Fear was a big factor. Fear was very big.

Richard: How did you deal with that?

Kathy Combs: Well, I just denied that I needed it and decided that "Hey, the next best thing is going to be out there because I'm going to wait for that." Because to do that implant, that's irreversible. Once you do that, there is no turning back. You've changed the functionality of your [crosstalk 00:10:59].

Richard: Did you talk about residual hearing it all, retaining residual hearing? Did you have any feelings about that?

Kathy Combs: I did have some residual hearing. However, when I had my surgery, what was very interesting is, my surgeon told me that there really wasn't much. I thought there was and after the surgery I realized that there was some. For example, the ceiling fan. I remember hearing that at night. The house was quiet, there was no other ambient noise, but I could hear the ceiling fan, and after the surgery, I didn't hear it. He also said, "People that have some residual hearing, I give them steroids," I believe, "to help preserve." And he said that, "In your case I wouldn't because there's not much there."

Richard: So, you consulted the surgeon, you scheduled for a cochlear implant. Do you remember how many months down the road from the time you decided to do it until the time you had surgery?

Kathy Combs: When I finally did see the surgeon... I met with him and on the first appointment he said to me, "You're definitely a candidate." And he also said to me, "And I would recommend Cochlear Americas as the branch." And I said, "Well, don't I get a choice?" He said, at that time in 2016, prior to the surgery, at that time Cochlear America was the only company that had the hybrid. And his feeling was that while I needed the regular implant in the right ear, my left ear was a candidate for the hybrid.

Richard: So, you didn't do the hybrid at the time?

Kathy Combs: Not yet.

Richard: So, you did your left ear [crosstalk 00:12:46].

Kathy Combs: Actually, I did my right ear.

Richard: You did your right ear with a regular cochlear implant?

Kathy Combs: Exactly.

Richard: And you left your left ear for the future, if you need it, is that correct?

Kathy Combs: Correct, correct.

Richard: Okay.

Kathy Combs: So, that's where I am today.

Richard: And you go to the hospital for surgery that day and you're still a little bit scared?

Kathy Combs: Yeah.

Richard: Tell me about the surgery a little bit. What happened after?

Kathy Combs: I was anxious about the surgery. However, the staff, it was a surgery clinic at Tampa, the staff there I just cannot say enough about. They were probably used to... Because I think that place, all they did were ENT type surgeries, and probably primarily cochlear implants. They were very familiar with the process. I think they answered multiple questions for me, they did whatever they could to ease my anxiety and make me feel more comfortable.

Kathy Combs: Next thing I knew I'm getting the intravenous sedative, and this was after my surgeon had spoken to me as well, so I felt like everybody had talked to me. And prior to the surgery, of course, there are a couple pre-op type visits in Tampa because you need to do the testing, and all those times the surgeon did speak to me as well, I believe, or at least twice before the surgery,

Richard: The surgeon, in this case, was one who recommended the brand. I ask this question because many people who are just investigating getting an implant, they get what we call a document dump, where the audiologist dumps all the brochures on, you're forced to decide, which is probably one of the most confusing parts. But in your case the surgeon recommended which you get.

Kathy Combs: Well, interesting, the audiologist who did the testing before I saw the surgeon, that evaluation period, had shown me the three different types, and the pluses, the minuses, pros, and cons.

Kathy Combs: And she basically said, "So, these are your choices." And I thought, "Well, how do I make a decision?" But then as soon as I saw the surgeon, he was the one who said to me, "I would suggest Cochlear America for you based on what's going on in the right ear, and some of the hearing you have in the left."

Kathy Combs: Because I'm indecisive, that was very helpful for me.

Richard: You made your choice. Do you have any regrets about what you've chosen?

Kathy Combs: No.

Kathy Combs: I think the only partial regret is that I was implanted with Nuclear 6. Within six months, there was the Nucleus 7. So, I'm with the slightly older technology until four more years pass.

Richard: That happens.

Kathy Combs: That happens.

Richard: Yes, it's [crosstalk 00:15:53]. That's a legitimate regret, but that's just timing. That's what we call the red line, "Just didn't know." What happened since? Was there any feature of the 6, or the accessories you like in particular?

Kathy Combs: Well, since it's my first one, and I have no other basis for comparison, obviously the clarity of sound I really like. I like the ease of programming. I have a remote and I use that for programming.

Richard: It changed your life how?

Kathy Combs: It made me become less isolated. I remember prior to the surgery, November, and December 2016 because I did not want to do the surgery prior to holidays, and so forth. I just remember that feeling of such isolation. We had had Thanksgiving together with some neighbors and it was just hard for me to follow the conversations. Just like somebody mentioned at the meeting, you're afraid to say anything because you feel like, "Are we still on that topic? Did somebody change the topic? Or did somebody say what I wanted to say already?"

Richard: You had your cochlear implant, it had been activated, do you still have that feeling from time to time?

Kathy Combs: Sometimes because it's not perfect. It's not restored, for me, normal hearing and just having the one ear, we are bilateral hearing.

Richard: Bimodal, bimodal.

Kathy Combs: Bimodal. So, I think the amount of input I'm getting from this hearing aid, I think it maxed out.

Richard: What do you have on that side?

Kathy Combs: I still have an Oticon and my audiologist in Tampa had talked to me about the ReSound because it does work with Cochlear America. However, she did say to me, "I don't know how much more you might get based on the audiogram in your left ear; I don't know how helpful it will be, especially if you are thinking somewhere down the road about doing another implant."

Richard: All right. That's a very interesting topic because you thought about a second implants, obviously. Can you talk a little bit about what the pros and cons in your mind?

Kathy Combs: So, the con, I have several friends who are bilateral implant wearers and one that I've become close to has said to me, "I take them both off, I am completely deaf, and I have to deal with the fact that I am deaf and sometimes that's a little scary for me."

Richard: If you take your implant off now and you take your hearing aid off now?

Kathy Combs: I am deaf.

Richard: Okay. That's what I think people want to know about because so many people have to deal with the fact, they might get one. What's the second one going to be like? But in the future, you would consider getting a second one?

Kathy Combs: Yes. My surgery day friend, that I met the day of my surgery and have become close to, did have a second one, and she's thrilled. She is thrilled. And it was a much easier adjustment with the second one from what she has told me. It was very easy transition and I believe she had it... I think the surgeon had said to wait six months prior to having a second one. And I think she waited about that amount of time, maybe a little bit longer. Now I don't remember the exact date, but she's very happy with it.

Richard: I'd like to go back to vocations again, for the moment.

Kathy Combs: Mm-hmm (affirmative).

Richard: You spoke about your career and the hearing loss. Then, when you lost your hearing, you were already retired. Have you found any other vocation you'd like to go into now? Or have you got a change that you got your implant?

Kathy Combs: Well, I'm very fortunate in that I am still working as a nurse. I work for a company that does testing. They test people who want to become certified nursing assistants. So that testing requires that people who apply for this, or apply to take the test, must do both the written tests and a clinical skills test. So, another nurse and I are in a room that mimics maybe an assisted living place, and we watch these two people, one takes care of the other, and we evaluate whether they're meeting the skills, the checkpoints.

Richard: In other words, you must be able to hear everything they're saying?

Kathy Combs: Exactly.

Richard: And can you?

Kathy Combs: I can, better than I ever could. I will tell you what is challenging, people with accents because we do probably have 25% of people that have accents. So, accents are a little challenging. I can sometimes adjust the remote, I can bump the volume up. People especially who speak very quietly because they're very nervous, I find sometimes even the other nurse will say, "Could you speak up please? I need to give your credit for what you're saying."

Richard: In other words, people with normal hearing or having problems in the same situation?

Kathy Combs: Exactly, exactly.

Richard: But you function to very high level now that you've had a cochlear implant, in a way you couldn't have before, right?

Kathy Combs: Exactly. And I'm also doing, I work for Manatee Technical College and do first aid and CPR classes, and that was a little challenging too because here's a group and you're the instructor. I generally always tell them ahead of time that I do have a hearing loss and I may have to ask you to repeat if you're going to ask a question. But most of the time it seems to not be a big problem, so I'm very happy to be able to do that.

Richard: Isn't that great? Are we thrilled? Are we...? Yeah.

Kathy Combs: Yeah. Very happy to be able to do that as well.

Richard: My last two questions are about music. Do you listen to music?

Kathy Combs: I do listen to music, but music is still a challenge. I do find the music I'm most comfortable with is music that I knew before.

Richard: Is that right?

Kathy Combs: Yeah. Older music or music that I can mentally [crosstalk 00:00:22:14].

Richard: Did you have to learn to hear music again, or does it come back... Why? Because you have a hearing aid on one side?

Kathy Combs: It is more challenging that I can't always follow the rhythm. Like if I'm in a situation, say for example in a church setting, and people are singing, I'm not always sure I'm on key, I'm not. Music has been a challenge.

Richard: And if you're in a church setting, is there a T-coil in your church or...?

Kathy Combs: Yes, yes.

Richard: So that brings the sound right to your processor?

Kathy Combs: Well, only if the people singing are singing through a microphone, but they're usually not, so that doesn't help.

Richard: Are there any features you would like to see that you don't have on the cochlear implant? I know you're waiting for the N7 because it has a few more features.

Kathy Combs: Mm-hmm (affirmative).

Richard: But what would you like to see that... You don't know?

Kathy Combs: Well, I have several of the portable features. I purchased the accessories like the microphone. I have found the microphone is a great, great accessory for me.

Richard: How do you use the microphone at home?

169

Kathy Combs: I tend to use it more in the car. Today, I picked up my daughter from Tampa airport. She speaks fast, she speaks softly. I clip the microphone, not actually onto her, but onto something that was close to her. I think on seatbelt because if it's too close, it's too much sound, what I found. And I was shocked, I was able to hear her conversation for the whole ride. That, to me, is huge. I used to not be able to hear her in the car or understand her. I knew she was saying something, so I could hear some noise, but I could not understand. So, for me, that has been huge. We just didn't talk in the car.

Richard: Now that you have your hearing back, with the sound back, do you have any goals for the future you'd like to do that you could not have conceived of before?

Kathy Combs: Well, I don't think I want to climb Everest anymore because that just seems just way too dangerous, so that's off the table. Just to continue to improve right now what I have, and to optimize what I have in terms of other long-range goals. I'm trying to practice being better with the phone. I will tell you the phone is sometimes still of a challenge for me.
Richard: How are you using the phone clip with the phone?

Kathy Combs: The phone clip has gotten better since my last audiology appointment. I was struggling with the Phone Clip. My last appointment the audiologist adjusted the settings and it's much better, it is much better. I really think that was a piece of it. I find using the Phone Clip with my cell phone, I understand better than the captioned phones. Captioned phone isn't as clear as it used to be to me. I must turn the volume way up, so working on improving being able to do the phones.

Richard: That's fabulous. I'm going to thank you for your time, but before we end, I just wanted to ask, do you have any advice for others who might be sitting on the fence?

Kathy Combs: I have a family member, a lovely sister, who helped get me to where I am today. She's right through the Peer Mentor Program at Gallaudet University and she's younger than I am, so I feel that we discussed this. There's probably some genetic predisposition in our family. She has not been ready yet to do this and I hope she will continue, and I hope other people who are considering this will continue to research it, and maybe feel some comfort level with being able to move forward because you're missing a lot.

Richard: I know this is hearsay, but do you know why she does not want to move forward, or you just guess?

Kathy Combs: I'm not sure if she's waiting for maybe the next new technology that isn't so permanent, I suppose. I'm not sure. She's wellversed on the surgery. She sent me information from her course. She spoke to, and heard from, so many experts through that program. She just couldn't say enough about it. Plus, it was long, it was two years. So, it's not lack of knowledge. I think there's some hesitation, possibly some fear.

Richard: I hope if she comes to visit you here, she'll sit down for an interview with me. I would be very interested to find out about that.

CHAPTER 13 SUZANNE TILLOTSON

A BILATERAL COCHLEAR IMPLANT NURSE IN THE COVID ICU SECTION

I recently came across this post on social media. It stopped me in my tracks, and I knew I had to have Suzanne Tillitson's story as part of the library of podcasts on Cochlear Implant Basics.

There seems to be nothing that can stop Suzanne from accomplishing her goals. She is an ICU nurse with bilateral cochlear implants. Cochlear implants made much of it possible but her amazing perseverance and dedication is inspirational.

This is her story:

Hi everyone! I hope you all are doing well. The bilateral CI life is treating me well. My word recognition is at 98% bilaterally and if we weren't masked (double and triple ply) I'd be able to understand most anything. Do I still practice? Absolutely!

What is my best story since I've become bilateral? Well, it's a sad story. I'm all about the positive, but there are some sad things my implants have allowed me to do.

This year has been difficult for all involved. It's been especially difficult on patients hospitalized with COVID and their caregivers.

Most recently I cared for a person at the end of life. The family was snowed in several hours away. I clocked out, set up the video monitor and called the family. My Eko stethoscope was gingerly placed where I could hear my friend's heartbeat while I sat nearly under the bed and held the hand of a dying father while his daughter cried and said "Dad, I'm holding your hand." I'd squeeze his hand to let him know he was not alone. "I'm with you Dad. I'm singing your favorite song Daddy. You are my sunshine, my only sunshine." All the while I held his hand. I stayed tucked under the view of the video in hopes the family didn't feel I was intrusive.

The heartbeat slowed, breathing slowed to a few breaths a minute and their father passed away peacefully holding my hand as proxy to his daughter.

My implants made this possible. My implants allowed me to return to my job as a nurse. My implants allowed me to be uprooted and deployed (I don't like this term) to another hospital and begin the life of a COVID nurse. My implants allowed me the honor of hearing the last heartbeats of the loneliest people in the world. They provided me with hope for a better future for myself and now I work to provide a better future for our families and those recovering from COVID.

Never sell yourself short. Being deaf doesn't define me or limit me. It made me a better nurse, mother, and wife. The implants gave me the ability to communicate properly and effectively. If you are ever having doubts, think of me. If I can do this every day. Anyone can. Much love to you all in your journey.

Suzanne Tillotson: My name is Suzanne Tillotson, I go by Susan. I'm in Greenville, South Carolina, and it is May 10th, 2021.

Richard Pocker: Now tell me a little bit about your hearing loss, how did it occur, how old were you, and so on and so forth? I'm going to let you have the floor.

Suzanne Tillotson: I have Meniere's disease. I've had Meniere's disease probably from a very, very young age. Because my mother tells me that I would have dizzy spills, and spin and fall, and my brother would hold me, and help me, and try to calm me down, because I was always scared. I didn't start having hearing loss though, until my late twenties. It was very, very mild. Everyone said don't worry about it. I worked for an ophthalmologist, who didn't really believe that it was real, and that the Meniere's disease was a thing. So, it prolonged me getting help because I really believed in everything she said. But a little bit later, when I started having more vertigo, I got to the point where I could not walk. I could not function. I was dizzy all the time, throwing up all the time. And, I met a doctor named Habib Rizk, and he determined that it was in fact, Meniere's.

Suzanne Tillotson: I had been diagnosed by a local EMT, who didn't know anything about Meniere's, but didn't know anybody to refer me to either, at the time. Dr. Rizk, however, he studied Meniere's disease in Lebanon. And it was a passion of his, that he was going to come to the United States, and he was going to take control of this. And, my husband took me to my medical doctor, carried me in, and said, fix her. And the medical doctor, standing there with his mouth open, going, oh, well I can't, but we'll find you someone who can. And they sent me to Charleston. I, that was six years ago. So, through treatment to get my balance back, we also started working on my hearing. So, he tried hearing aids for a little while. They did not work. My vertigo got worse. I had an endolymphatic sac decompression, and shortly after my recovery from that, I got hit by a patient, and it destroyed the ear. So then, I had to have a labyrinthectomy. And that was my first experience with a cochlear implant.

Richard Pocker: Did they do it simultaneously?

Suzanne Tillotson: No, they did it a year apart, because I had other physical damage. That one's hard to talk about, but I had broken nose, lost teeth. There was a lot.

Richard Pocker: Because, we have one other interview with Meniere's patient, and she had the labyrinthectomy and the cochlear implant done, simultaneously. So, you're in a different situation.

Suzanne Tillotson: That's normal. That is normally how that would be done. But, since I had other damage, and I couldn't walk, and there was so much to it, I couldn't even talk. There was a lot to that.

Richard Pocker: And, had the one done. How was the rehab when you had the first one done?

Suzanne Tillotson: Well, I was very, very dedicated to vestibular therapy. So, when I knew that this was going to happen, I knew the surgery was going to happen. I've just hunkered down, and did the vestibular therapy with the PT offices, and then I learned a way to do it at home, by myself. So, I modified their therapy, to fit a one-person therapy, and did it all, every day. I mean, an hour every morning, every day, to where I got to work, I'd walk straight, everything. If I left my labyrinthectomy the day I had it done, most people stay in the hospital a couple of days, and I left. We ate dinner after, and it was a four-hour drive. We stopped halfway, and I ate dinner, and he tells me, that it's because I did all the vestibular therapy before. It is terrifying, because the explanation of the surgery was that it was going to be difficult, I'm going to be very ill after, if I'm up at all, I'm going to rely on a walker. I did use a cane, for a little while.

Richard Pocker: Okay. And your hearing when you got the cochlear implant, describe that, the activation.

Suzanne Tillotson: See, I wasn't expecting anything, because I was still hurt. I was still internally hurt, by the whole thing. So, I wasn't expecting really great things. The day I got activated from my cochlear implant, on the drive home, he called me and asked me how I was feeling. I had already hooked it up to my phone. I was playing with it. So, I had already hooked it up to my phone, and was trying to hear little dots, and beeps, and everything. Well, he called on my phone and I answered it. But I answered it with my cochlear implant, I didn't realize it. And we had a full conversation through my cochlear implant the day I was activated, and I said, I'm hearing you through it now, I can't believe this. And I was able to have a full conversation. Words, like we would be having right now, because I'm not connected to the computer, or harder for me, that took rehab. So, I've used this ear only, I've read out loud, I've listened to old music that I grew up listening to, which in my case, it's Elvis, because that's when my mother loved. It was just great. That's how I did my rehab. I did my rehab, he told me I overdid everything. I'm his all-in girl.

Richard Pocker: I think the lesson learned here, is the fact that when rehabilitation takes place, you can't make it wrong. You just must be dedicated to doing it. You can't expect it to happen overnight. You had a rock star activation.

Suzanne Tillotson: I did. I had a rock star activation, and he tells me that, because when I got my other ear done, he told me not to expect it to be like the first one.

Richard Pocker: Well, that's a very good point. Tell me about the second one. How did that go?

Suzanne Tillotson: The second one was, the past October a year ago. So, 2020, I had sudden hearing loss in the right ear. For about a week, I heard a high pitch roar, and then it was gone. It was nothing. It was scary, horrifying. And it was from an activation of the Meniere's, on that side. And then the trauma that I had previously, he says associated with that. I knew right away; I want a cochlear implant. There's no second guessing that.

Richard Pocker: Did the same surgeon do the second one?

Suzanne Tillotson: Oh yes.

Richard Pocker: Which hospital?

Suzanne Tillotson: MUSC at Charleston. Medical University of South Carolina.

Richard Pocker: Was the second activation as good, was the first, or?

Suzanne Tillotson: It didn't come off without a hitch, like the first one. I chose a different mode. I have an N7 on this side, but it wasn't, right here. Since the N7 is more flexible, I put it on the ear that I had a little flexibility with. With this ear, I have no flexibility, because I had a labyrinthectomy. So, I can't do different things with it, because of that.

Suzanne Tillotson: I ended up with a Kanso over here, which is what I originally chose for this year. With the Kanso, they put it on, I was immediately disappointed when they activated it, because it was Alvin and the Chipmunks, that's all I could hear. And before, I didn't have the Alvin and the Chipmunks sound. This time, it was nothing but Alvin and the Chipmunks. Everyone sounded like it. And I was just waiting on Dave to talk, Simon, and Theodore, and Dave.

Suzanne Tillotson: I was depressed for a few days because it was so different. But I took off my processor over here, and I started reading out loud, I started listening to the music. I started doing everything that I'm supposed to do, that I didn't on the other ear. It took twice as long. I did not have any vertigo with the surgery, because of the rehab that I do every day. But it took a lot longer. But now, I mean, it's not even been a year that I've had this implant. So, I can take this one off, and function perfectly over here. Because that's still considered a part of the rehab for it.

Richard Pocker: Would you ever get another N7 for the other ear, at some point?

Suzanne Tillotson: For this side? No, I like the Kanso. I get better sound quality out of this ear. I don't know why there's a difference, but I still get better sound quality over here.

Richard Pocker: It's interesting, because I like to use the phrase, no two hearing losses are exactly the same. Those individuals are fingerprints, and the rehabilitation's the same way. And you've shown that with two different modes of cochlear implants, that you can still function very well. I'd like to ask you a little bit more about your career, and how the cochlear implant had an effect, on what you do. Talk more about what you do for work, and your life.

Suzanne Tillotson: I'm a nurse. I've been a nurse for almost 19 years. And I thought that my hearing loss was going to end my career. And most people did. Most people go into this, thinking that they're [inaudible 00:10:20]. I talk to people online all the time who think, okay, I'm not going to be working anymore. And I'm always like, no, you keep going. You keep trying, you keep working and you can do it. So being a nurse, we use stethoscopes that go inside the ear. They don't work because you can't hear. So, I use an Eko, an Eko CORE, and it transmits through my processors, now. That's a new thing they have. It normally would go through your phone, and then go to your ears. But now, I compare my stethoscope with my processors. But the last year, since COVID hit, they call it deployed.

Suzanne Tillotson: I'd never considered us fighting in the army, being in the war. But we were taken from a hospital that was for med surge, appendectomies, gallbladder surgery. I see you have your surgery. I make sure you're good. You eat, you drink, you go to the bathroom. You go home. I liked that. I liked seeing that progress, that you do. When we were brought over to this other hospital, I see people who are sick and dying, and they can't breathe. They're struggling. And the only way I can do my job, is because I have my implants. Because I would not be able to hear them breathe. I would not be able to hear their hearts beat. I would not be able to listen to their fears, or at the beginning, be their mother, sister, daughter, niece. You must be everything for that patient. And if I should not hear them properly, I would not be able to do it at all.

Richard Pocker: But you were able to do with the cochlear implant?

Suzanne Tillotson: Yes, absolutely.

Richard Pocker: That brings me to a very interesting point, because I read recently about, I believe the pronunciation is, auscultation, The ability to hear the heartbeat, or hear through the cochlear implant. The internal sounds are so critical, that if you don't hear them exactly right, you may not be functioning properly. You may not get the right diagnosis. Could you talk a little bit about how you hear through the stethoscope?

Suzanne Tillotson: At first it was through my phone, and then it was sent from my phone to my ears. So, I trained myself, while I was out. I had downloaded videos of normal heart sounds, and I listened to those through my stethoscope, for several weeks. Then, I started listening to abnormal heart tones, and now I'm proficient. I'm more proficient now, than I was, before I had my surgery. Before I lost my hearing, because I didn't put this much time into learning normal and abnormal heart tones, before I lost my hearing. But I was determined that you're going to know what you're doing, because you're not going to screw this up. So now, I have this Eko stethoscope that I can unhook, and put on a person's chest with enough pressure. I can be doing something else, while I'm listening to their heartbeat. So, especially if they're asleep, and I can listen to their rhythms, and I can listen to that heartbeat.

Suzanne Tillotson: And especially if a patient is not doing well, and is going to pass away, and you can listen to their heartbeat, and hear that, okay, they're not progressing, this is going to be the day. I need to prepare their family. But I had to train myself first. So, I downloaded audio recordings of normal, abnormal, all of it, while I was out on leave. That's what I learned to do.

Richard Pocker: You're unbelievable. You are a total inspiration. People are going to listen to this and understand. I hope that having a cochlear implant makes you unstoppable.

Suzanne Tillotson: Well, I've been unstoppable, so far. The only time that it catches me off guard, is when I lean against, say metal, wall, or door jam, and this one flies off my head. And then I'm like, I've dropped it. And you crawl around on your hands and knees, thinking you dropped it, and there it is, all [inaudible 00:14:32] because the magnet is so strong.

Richard Pocker: How many people have left it on their car doors, drive away, find it at the other end of the ride?

Suzanne Tillotson: This happened at a nail salon. And I stopped this lady from getting in her car, because I didn't know where it went. And I'm on my hands and knees, and she needs to leave. And I'm sorry lady, but if I lose my implants, I'm toast. So, you're going to have to wait. It was on her car door. I had a lot of fun with my implants, because there's a lot of stimulation that people must get used to, especially when you're bimodal. Once you have bilateral hearing, all this extra sound comes in, that you haven't been used to for a long time.

Suzanne Tillotson: And in my world, it's very loud in my family, and my work, and everything. It's all very loud. You must unplug, sometimes. And after a major event at work, at first, it's loud, and it's hard to concentrate on one person, when it's loud, especially when we're wearing two masks, head gear, all this gowns, and everything. And you can only hear the movement of your gown. And you're trying to focus on a doctor. At the end of that, I would go in a little room, and take off both of my processors, just sit there, and unplug for just a few minutes, because there was so much stimulation. That was a challenge for me.

Richard Pocker: I hear that all the time, that I'm overstimulated. I need to take a break. Everybody's different. And including the scan programs on your individual processors, people like different ways of hearing.

Suzanne Tillotson: If I'm having an emergency, I click my phone, I change it to a different program, and it's, Forward Focus is what I use, so I could hear the doctor, only. And it helps knock out everybody behind me. And I can run that code with my doctor, and I can hear him better, or her better. Whoever's giving the orders. I know how to run a code, but you must wait and see, what this doctor wants to do next.

Richard Pocker: Yeah. One thing I'd love to talk to about, was because your hearing loss was relatively late, relatively sudden. Talk to me a little bit about your coworkers. The doctors you work with, the other nurses who work with, were they cooperative? Was a problem? They knew you had an issue.

Suzanne Tillotson: Yes, I was very clear, because I had to get a new job after I was injured. So, I came into this job that I have now. I was so open about it, that I wanted her, the person that I was going to work for, who I didn't know I was going to get this job with, I am deaf. I'm going to have other surgeries because I hadn't had my right ear done yet. And I needed her to understand, that at this point, I'm not normal yet. I'm going to be, but I'm not there yet. And I was still having some episodes of the dizziness. And at first, it took her by surprise that I was so honest about it. She hired me on the spot. Because when I left the other hospital, I was devastated. Like two weeks, I was devastated. Didn't do anything. And then, I put it on resume, and I got 23 phone calls in 48 hours. That changed my whole world. I went with one interview for a place that I wanted to go. And she hired me on the spot, and it changed my life.

Richard Pocker: Talk a little bit about your future. I understand you're going through more studies for advancement. Tell us what you're doing, and where are you going to be?

Suzanne Tillotson: Well, I think I'm going to end up finishing it in Clemson, which Clemson University, is where I got my bachelor's degree in Nursing, because I started out slow. I got my Associates Degree, worked as a nurse, went back, got my bachelor's degree. Worked as a nurse, was getting my Master's, my Nurse Practitioner's License, when I got injured and had to stop, because I could not do all of it. I could not get well. I focused on getting well and do that too. It was a lot. So, I'm going back, but I'm going to do Nursing Administration and Leadership, because I want to be a leader on the field. I want to be the person that says, yes, you can do this, but you're going to have to work at it. Because that comes in nursing too. You don't walk in out of school and know how to do everything.

Suzanne Tillotson: You know the basic function of life, but you don't know the basic function of how a hospital operates, or the machinery. And I want to be the person that helps those people. You can do this. I met a nurse who was losing her hearing, and she was just starting out. And she came in, and realized that she just couldn't hear well enough, to hear the heart sounds. And so now, she is getting a cochlear implant. So, it's like, this happened to me in a bad way. And then the injury and everything, had happened in a really, bad way. Also, [inaudible 00:19:46] for like a week. And then, all right, I'm done. Let's make this work for some other reason, this had to happen, so I could do something with it. And I've met several people now, who've had implants, because you can do this, and call me. I've got you. It's been nice. That's what I want to keep doing.

Richard Pocker: You never know who you're going to help. You never know what their future is going to be. You have a mission. I have a mission.

Suzanne Tillotson: You have a mission, yes, and love your mission.

Richard Pocker: We must talk to people, who are scared to death, that they've lost the hearing, scared to death about a cochlear implant, because they have misconceptions, brain surgery that it's going to sound mechanical. So, we both have a very parallel mission. And I really, really appreciate the time you spent with me, I'm sure your story is going to inspire others to move forward. Do you have anything you'd like to add before we close?

Suzanne Tillotson: Just that I'm glad to have met you and talk to you. I've read things that you've written, and what you've written to other people. And I think that your mission is so important to get this out there to everyone, because we are a minority. You don't realize it, until you experience it.

Richard Pocker: Thank you for being part of the same journey. I appreciate your time. I hope you have a chance to speak again soon, and we'll take care.

Chapter 14 Nanette Florian

Hear Music Again! Cochlear Implant Journey of a Lead Singer Who Lost Her Hearing

Many cochlear implant candidates are more concerned about music than speech.

When I learned about Nanette Florian's passion for helping fellow cochlear implant recipients and those with hearing loss get the best out of music, I knew I had to ask her to sit down for an interview.

She started playing the piano and singing when she was five years old.

She is a former member of The New Christy Minstrels, she was the standing bass and lead singer during her time with the group.

Eventually, her hearing declined to the point where she stopped playing. That was until she received a cochlear implant 14 years ago.

Today her outreach is through her website Hear Music Again hearmusicagain.org

Along with her brother John, who also suffers with a hearing loss, they have two internet radio stations WHMA (Hear Music Again) and WHRA (Hear Rock Again). They are an eclectic mix of genres that were selected not only for the clarity but variety. There is a wide range of rock, blues, and funky soul as well as soft rock and country and classical music.

Nanette Florian: My name is Nanette Florian. My location is Rhode Island on the ocean and the date is Tuesday, the 22nd of June 2021.

Richard: Thank you so much. I first like to start out asking you about the history of your hearing loss, how you discovered it, what steps you took. Tell me a little bit about your background.

Nanette Florian: My father, when I was growing up, he had very big hearing aids. He always said that it happened during the war. But I have two brothers and one of my other brothers and myself, when we turned about 19 or 20, we realized we had a hearing loss as well. It wasn't my father's, you know, not bombs falling and everything. He had bad hearing when he went into the war and then his hearing got worse. My brother and I started wearing hearing aids too. My two children have hearing aids. Obviously, it runs in the family. So, when I was 19 or so I got a little in the ear hearing aid and as time went on, by the time I reached 40, oh, I had big hearing aids. And about 15 years ago, I had cochlear surgery.

Richard: You've discovered your hearing loss was very profound by that time, obviously. Probably a little bit about the qualifications for your cochlear implant. You went to an ENT or audiologist. Tell me a little bit about that.

Nanette Florian: I'm trying to remember what happened. I think my audiologists that worked with me for the hearing aids, I think we realized they weren't working anymore, and I was fed up. But we didn't have the money to get the cochlear processor. After a lot of research, I found, I can't remember the name of the donation group in Colorado, and they donated the processor to me, and I have one. Just one processor. We had to pay for the surgery, but it was just delightful to have gotten the cochlear processor. It really works well.

Richard: So how long have you had it now?

Nanette Florian: Probably 14 years. And I still have the same.

Richard: What make of cochlear implant do you have?

Nanette Florian:

Cochlear Americas.

Nanette Florian:

Yeah, I have a Freedom, Nucleus Freedom. It's an oldie.

Richard: You're the first person I've spoken to who's still using the Freedom.

Nanette Florian:

Yeah. I'm into vintage things. Works well. I have two of them. And when I first got them, there seemed to be problems all the time. And I was always sending it back again and they would be sending me parts, which worked fine. But, for many years now nothing's happened. It's been great.

Richard: Let's knock on wood right here.

Nanette Florian: Yeah. Something's going to happen…

Richard: Let me ask you another question. You only have it on one side?

Nanette Florian: Yeah.

Richard: Are you wearing a hearing aid on the other?

Nanette Florian: Well, like I said, it, money was a struggle because we're self-employed and we didn't have insurance to cover it. We decided we were just happy that I had one side and it was such a huge improvement on my hearing that I thought, well, I don't need the other side. I understand the other side is important and you can hear a lot better. And another thing is, I like the idea of one ear, having nothing on it. After having these big hearing aids on my ears for so many years, I enjoy just having nothing on that ear. You know, feeling kind of normal on this side, but I don't know what's going to happen in my future. I may go for it. If I'm going to have to get new processors and I may have to go for the other side surgery too.

Richard: If you go to the other side, obviously they're going to upgrade the processor to something new. And if you go to a clinic that it's a twoprocessor clinic, you'll get one for each side. So, that's a possibility. Now the residual hearing you have on the one side; it doesn't have the implant. Is there any hearing at all there or not?

Nanette Florian: No, no, no. I can sleep through a thunderstorm. There's no hearing at all.

Richard: Yeah. I understand that feeling. I was deaf for 35 years before I got cochlear implants. I could sleep through anything.

Nanette Florian: Yeah. Do you have hearing aids then?

Richard: I wore hearing aids until I was 30. And then I lost all my residual hearing in a matter of weeks. I went totally silent for 35 years. And I only received cochlear implants just before my 65th birthday, but I received bilateral surgery. They did two sides at the same time. So, it's a little bit different. Now, I really would love to talk about your music career and how you hear music through them. If you could just give a little bit of background because I interviewed people who have been musically inclined, but not a professional like you. You know. I want to hear from your professional's point of view, after your career and how the hearing loss affected it and what you did.

Nanette Florian: I started playing the piano when singing, when I was five and there was this picture of Beethoven. Big, beautiful painting of Beethoven over the piano. I used to look up at him and go, oh, the poor guy lost his hearing. Never realizing that the same thing was going to

187

happen to me. But before it did, yes, I started out when I graduated from high school, I was, you know, involved in all kinds of music in high school. And my brother and I bought a motor home, and we did a musical duo and we traveled all over the country together, performing, deciding where we wanted to play, and it was just a fantastic time for two years. We were kind of like hippies, but not, not really. Then we got to California, and we tried out for the new Christy Minstrels and that was the late 1970s.

Nanette Florian: And they said, we'll call you, don't call us. And we traveled some more and performed some more, all over the place. And we were playing on Cape Cod in Massachusetts one summer and we had a phone call, and it was from Hollywood. And they wanted us to fly out in two days and be part of the new Christy Minstrels. So, I was the standup bass player. First female standup bass player for the new Christy Minstrels and a lead singer. And my brother played the guitar and sang. And we traveled with them for about a year, which was very difficult traveling all the time on a bus or, you know, whatever. And sometimes we would perform twice a day. It was tough. After that year, I went back to Connecticut where I'm originally from. And then I started my own solo career playing the piano and singing the Eastern seaboard.

Nanette Florian: And as time went on, I didn't want to play for people drinking anymore, the bars and all that, because I just didn't relate to the whole thing. So, I started becoming a worship team leader at church. And then I started realizing that I was singing off tune and these nice people at church didn't want to tell me that I was out of tune, but I was. And so that was all over with. Then as time went on, I couldn't even hear my own worship team. I couldn't hear the music at all. And actually, quit church because there was no sense in going in, you know. So, that's when I started searching out the cochlear processor. That was all hearing aid days. And then the processor just changed my life. I could hear on the phone again, and I could hear my family talking to me, and I could be a part of group conversations again, and it's been wonderful. But the only problem is that music is still distorted.

Richard: Distorted how? Can you give me a little bit more explicit description of how you heard music changing and how it came through with the cochlear implant? And did it get any better with time with your cochlear implant?

Nanette Florian: When I got my cochlear implant, I think because I am a musician, they told me that I caught on fast to sound. I started hearing very well quickly, but as far as music's concerned, it all sounds like it's kind of underwater and distorted to me. But occasionally, during those first days, I noticed that sometimes there was a song that would come through to me, nice and clearly. I decided that I can hear music, but I need to find it. I need to find the music that I can hear, because I know that there are sounds out there that I can hear. Like I noticed on your website, you had a gong or a kind of a bong chime thing that you put up. And that's exactly what I love the go for, is the chimes, I can hear them well and they vibrate too. You can feel it all the way through you. And that's a real sound. That's fun. You know, for us, people who don't get sound the way we should, like, you know, most people do.

Nanette Florian: What I've been doing now is collecting all this music. I've gone through thousands of songs to determine if I could hear them or not. And there's lots of recordings that are crisp and clear and easy to hear. I just needed to find them.

Richard: I think that's a fantastic idea. You know, the funny thing is when I got my hearing back after 35 years, I obviously missed 35 years of music. And I took a Sony Walkman to the local library and went through the CD collection by streaming the music through the accessory, to my cochlear implants. And that's how I caught up on 35 years of music.

Nanette Florian: Oh, good for you.

Richard: Which is very, very important for people to understand that if you get a cochlear implant, you may or may not recover all your music, but there are different techniques. What's the name of your website, by the way?

Nanette Florian: It's hearmusicagain.org

Richard: I'm going to make sure that people understand that and find that side as well. My next comment or question to you is because I have interviewed on the website, Jack Barnes, who was implanted 33 years ago, and he has gone through eight generations of processors. Perhaps it is a question that the Freedom is not as technically advanced, by the time you can upgrade to a Nucleus 7 or whatever you get at that time. Perhaps musical sound a lot better.

Nanette Florian: Yes. One thing I've noticed that men's voices dropped down a half a key. Like I'll be listening to a song, and I know what key it's in. I can hear it in my mind. And I know what the singer is supposed to sound like. You know, after the song has started, the singer starts up and the male voices, the beefier the voice, the lower, if he drops down and he's not singing in the same key as the instruments. That's something I've kind of noticed in higher voices. Like if it's a tenor, a man singing tenor, that he stays in key to me in most female voices stay in key to me as well. After I've collected all this music, I put it in internet radio stations. I have two radio stations. People like us can listen to 24 hours of music, seven days a week.

Richard: On your website?

Nanette Florian: Yep.

Richard: Okay. We were talking briefly before we had the interview, that when I was rehabilitating for music, I found that swing jazz was the easiest to rehabilitate to. When you were listening to music again, for the first time you do find something easier? Any genre of music you found more helpful to rehab with?

Nanette Florian: Yes. And I think like, you know, as well as a single instrument alone is great. When you start piling up too many instruments, they all sort of cancel each other out and turn into a bunch of mush. But jazz is great because the horns come through well to us. And you had a banjo player on your site, and I love the banjo. It comes through so well.

Richard: All those musicians I recruited, some of them did it for free. Some of them did it for $20 to give me a two-minute clip. And the only instrument I have not been able to get is harmonica. Harmonica players are the biggest pains in the...

Nanette Florian: Ah, they have attitude. Well, I wonder how the harmonica would come through. I've listened to harmonica music, and I wasn't sure that it was coming through clearly like a clarinet like Benny Goodman. I have such a good recording of Benny Goodman. There are only five guys in that particular recording. And so, we with hearing loss, we hear the rhythm, right? And then you can add a nice bass to that and that comes through pretty good. And then if you just add one more instrument to that, it's hearable. And especially if it's like a saxophone or a trumpet or a clarinet.

Richard: The acoustics fight with one another. And I understand exactly what you're talking about. I have a decent collection of Benny Goodman vinyl. I find vinyl. I can hear the difference in the warmth of vinyl versus CD. That's how good the Nucleus 7 is for me.

Nanette Florian: And the jazz players are great because they take turns. They're not always playing at the same time. On my radio stations, you're going to hear classical and jazz and oldies and authentic country. Not country that is played now because it's all full of reverb. All the music I try to get, you know, more modern songs on my radio shows, but there's too much reverb. So, I go back in time, even before reverb was used in recording, like Hank Williams at the Grand Old Opry. He was recording

191

live and there was no reverb and it's just him and his guitar. And it's fantastic. I have that in my playlist as well.

Richard: Each of us have a mission to help pay forward. Once we have a cochlear implant, we have a mission to pay it forward to help other people. You've done a fantastic job helping people with music because so many people I've spoken to are on the fence about getting a cochlear implant because they're afraid to lose music. Even if they have 10% hearing left, they want to hear music through a hearing aid, not a cochlear implant, but we do our best to help them get the best results. It's an ongoing thing. Rehabilitation never stops. It goes on for your life.

Nanette Florian: Right. Well, the people with the hearing aids, they've probably had music most of their lives like you and me. We know a lot of music. You get that back. Your brain picks it up again.

Richard: It takes time. Yes, but it does. It does. You know, one of the techniques I've found works very, very well. If you're trying to rehabilitate with songs that, you know, I send people to YouTube and tell them to add in the word, the name of the song with lyrics, because the brain sees the words and hears music and it works much, much faster that way.

Nanette Florian: Yeah. First, you need to know the name of the song you're listening to. And sometimes, you know, we'll be listening to music. There'll be a group of people. This was before my radio stations. Cause my radio stations, I hear everything very nicely and clearly. Maybe not intonation wise on the cochlear processor, melodies don't come through. But everything else is coming through. The processor is perfect for the spoken word, but it doesn't distinguish melodies, but it's still so much clearer. I'm so happy. I'm listening all the time to music, and I feel like my good old self. Again, I feel musical again.

Richard: Music's in your blood, it's in your genes.

Nanette Florian: Yes. And it's not good to miss out on it.

Richard: No, the socializing aspect of cochlear implants obviously are paramount. But music is in our genes. I mean, Tom Wolfe wrote a book recently called The Kingdom of Speech and in it he noted, even Darwin thought that people understood music before they spoke.

Nanette Florian: Oh yeah.

Richard: That's a very fascinating topic. And I'm just happy just to hear music again. I mean I stream all day long.

Nanette Florian: I am debuting my radio stations at the Hearing Loss Association of America's convention this weekend.

Richard: That's great.

Richard: I would like to ask you to take the floor, and if you have a message for people who are on the fence about getting a cochlear implant, what would you tell them?

Nanette Florian: I would say that the cochlear implant takes the stress away. It's so much clearer because I wore the hearing aids for all those years. And it was just so stressful. And the cochlear implant just brings it so deeply and sharply into your, you know, your brain and it just so much better, so much better than the hearing aids. It just so much sharper. I have a brother with hearing aids who has a moderate to profound, and he's on the fence about the cochlear processor too. And I know that I hear better than him.

Richard: That's very funny because I have another interview with a woman named Janet Fox, whose brother also has profound, very, very profound loss. She was the first to get the cochlear implant. I believe she was first. He was second. Then she got bilateral and then she was working on him to go bilateral. When you have a genetic loss, it's a different situation because you want the best for your spouses or siblings. And sometimes they're just stubborn and there's nothing you can do. But you keep working on him. And I appreciate your time. This is a wonderful interview. I'm sure people are going to enjoy it. I'll be sure that I mentioned your website, and I look forward to talking to you again sometime in the future.

Nanette Florian:

All right. Thank you. It was nice to meet you.

Chapter 15 Michelle M. Wagner

Mom of a Pediatric Cochlear Implant Recipient Who Stared Down Adversity and Won

If adversity is a test of character, Michelle Wagner has passed with flying colors. Deciding to adopt a child, a process that took a year, it was later discovered this beautiful baby had a profound hearing loss.

The doctors recommended bilateral cochlear implant surgery. This required a staggering amount of research and support, all which Michelle handled with aplomb while dealing with an impending divorce.

Faced with the choice of whether her son should go the route of sign language or mainstream with hearing, she decided on cochlear implants.

The road was not easy. Her son lacked any language skill, and he was three when he received his surgery. Her story is a true testament to perseverance and love. Today Mickey is a thriving thirteen-year-old.

Michelle M. Wagner: Hi, I'm Michelle Wagner, and I'm in Washington right now, and it's June 20th, 2021.

Richard: Thank you for joining me. I'd like to know a little bit more about your son, how you discovered he had a hearing problem, and I'm going to let you have the floor and tell me some background to it.

Michelle M. Wagner: Thank you, Richard. So, my ex-husband and I always wanted to be parents and we decided to adopt. And I have cousins in Ohio that had just adopted from Russia, so we decided to take that route. We adopted a beautiful little boy from Russia, and we brought him home. And two months after we were home, we realized... He was about 18 months, and we thought at first it was a language barrier, but it turned out that it didn't seem like he was hearing us. And we were banging pots and pans and he was just not turning around, and so we went to a local ENT. They put hearing aids on him. There didn't seem to be much of a change, and then we went straight to a larger hospital, a bigger audiology team and so forth, and they suggested bilateral cochlear implants. And so, it had to go through the FDA approval and all these other hoops to jump through. And Mickey was implanted at age three.

Richard: That and he had both done at the same time?

Michelle M. Wagner: Yes. We were fortunate enough for him to do bilateral cochlear implants in both ears at the same time.

Richard: Now three years old is considered a little bit older than most pediatrics, but how was his language development?

Michelle M. Wagner: At the time he had no language. He was just making sounds. And then after he was implanted, and of course, after the recovery period, it was still quite a challenge because it was his first-time hearing anything. We had started some sign language, and then after he was implanted, we had specialists talk to us and they said, "Do you want a speaking child? Or a signing child?" And we said, "Well, we have the cochlear implants. We want a speaking child." And there was a lot of different opinions, but the best thing that I did, or we did, for my son was, there was a special program in Southern California called the John Tracy Clinic, and it immerses you for about a month, the parents, and the children.

My son and I did this program.

Michelle M. Wagner: We lived in the dorm rooms there that they gave us, and it really showed us how to live with somebody with hearing impairments, with those challenges, and to be able to give him all the tools he needs. And to this day, we still, he needs to ask for something, he repeats it until he says it correctly. We got divorced during the time of his waiting for the operation, operation, et cetera, being implanted, and he had to go to special schooling, and the two of us just lived together. And that was probably the best thing to happen, and I had to change my life. I'm kind of a foodie with a restaurant background and there was no more going to restaurants.

Michelle M. Wagner: He needed the quiet environment of being at home, just the two of us, to not have the background noise, especially in the beginning. Special school, private speech aside from the special school. And then I wanted him to not feel any different and I wanted him to have confidence and he played sports. Other than the first two schools he was at, so up until about fourth grade, he did everything with other typical children. And until this day, he is 13 now.

Michelle M. Wagner: He finally went mainstream to a regular public school where we live, and now he's in a farm school. And until this day, he is confident. He is athletic. We are still going to speech three times a week, and it's always going to be a challenge. We're very positive. He has a great attitude. I couldn't ask for any better situation than, he hears and he's grateful.

Richard: Attitude plays so much a part in this because some parents are in an absolute panic, and after their child received cochlear implants, they still haven't calmed down. You've given a message that's very important for parents to know how important positive thinking is to get the best results.

Michelle M. Wagner: Absolutely.

Richard: Now, tell me a little bit about the auditory training he gets. Does he still go for training three times a week?

Michelle M. Wagner: Yes. He still goes to a private speech therapist just to work on sounds and expressive. He also has some other delays cognitively with learning, but he is a brilliant boy, very brilliant. He's a builder. He's very hands-on. He loves animals. He's an animal whisper. We have chickens at home, and he has... there at school, there's goats, and there's chickens, and bunnies. He loves all that. And the one thing, always in any school, or anyone that meets him, or is in school with him, Mickey is very empathetic.

Richard: I need to take you back a few steps because parents who find out their child has severe hearing loss, they're in a panic. Could you talk a little bit about when you met the surgeon, how you were feeling? What was going on in your head at that time when you met with the surgeon, and you knew your son had a problem?

Michelle M. Wagner: Yes. I was scared, yet I was willing to do whatever it took to give this boy every opportunity within my reach. And we had friends in the medical industry, we asked for opinions, did research, read everything. There are parent groups online that you could find that really put me at ease. It took a whole year to do the adoption, and that was a roller coaster.

Michelle M. Wagner: Then we finally get this beautiful boy, and then find out he cannot hear and speak. And it was devastating, but we were like, "Okay, what do we do?" And we find the best possible solution for this. And yes, at that same time, my then husband decided he didn't want to be married anymore, and there was a bunch of challenges. But now I look back and I don't know how we got through it, but-

Richard: You should be proud of what you got through. You should be very, very proud, because a lot of parents just don't know what to do. They collapse. And you didn't collapse for one second.

Michelle M. Wagner: No. We just wanted to do everything. And still until this day, I have his dad's support, and support in the community, and from everyone, just embracing this.

Richard: How did you find the support? That's an important question. How did you find the people that would help support you?

Michelle M. Wagner: Well, support, I think emotionally supportive is what I'm... and family and friends. I'm fortunate enough to always have family and friends. And I was always the helper, and I was the oldest child. I thought I had everything together, and for the first time in life, multiple things were... it was a domino effect of me needing to ask for help. And that's the thing that every parent, or a person that's going to be a cochlear recipient needs to know. Ask for help because the help is out there. Emotional help is out there. There's financial help there.

Michelle M. Wagner: And if you just go into a shell... And the last thing for small children that I knew I didn't want to do is act like it was an issue, make it a problem. I wanted my son to know and to feel that he is 100% loved. He is 100% a normal child. He can do anything he wants, and mom and dad are strong and supportive. And because he has felt safe from day one, he's taken it all in stride. And most recently, I released a book about him as an elementary student trying to tell others about his cochlear implants, because a lot of people don't know what they are. And it's been a huge success. And the whole point of it is awareness and education. Education is what everything comes down to.

Richard: I had that discussion almost every single day, that education is the biggest problem of all. And so many doctors don't even know what a cochlear implant is. The public has no idea. It's a constant struggle for the education, and what I hear from you is you are paying it forward by educating other people. Even by doing this video, you'll probably reach five or 600 people next week, and somebody's going to click and say, "Thank you for making the video. Thank you for explaining what's going on." Let me ask you another question. Since he was so young, do you remember what activation day was like when they turned him on? Can you tell me about that?

Michelle M. Wagner: They told us it might be very scary or traumatic, and they activated him, and he just seemed happier. And it was actually a good experience. I know for a lot of adults, it's more emotional, and for people that have heard before, I think that it's different, and maybe some of them do not like how it sounds. But for my son, it was the first time ever he was hearing. And just like you have the Nucleus 7 now, that's what he has as well. And he started out with the Nucleus 5 and then 6. And he hears whispers. He lets us know if something's too loud or not loud enough. And we meet with his audiologist now only once a year for mapping and things like that. Medicine is so amazing, and the doctors, and the technology that's out there incredible. And they came up with, not too many years ago, Cochlear's Aqua. He can swim with his friends. Being 13, it's important, and that's amazing.

Richard: Parents that I've spoken to are sometimes torn about getting a cochlear implant because they're afraid their child's speech will never sound normal. Can you tell me a little bit about Mickey's speech? I know he's still going to training, but tell me objectively, what do you think his speech sounds like?

Michelle M. Wagner: Those of us that are around him all the time, he's easy to understand. I do want you and everyone who's listening to keep in mind that Mickey does have some other cognitive delays, so that the comprehension of the speech... But receptively, it's amazing. And his speech, he doesn't sound like you would expect. He does not sound like he is deaf. He sounds-

Richard: Like the deaf speech. The accent.

Michelle M. Wagner: Right. And he sounds like he has cochlear implants and perhaps some vocabulary issues. But overall, it's also a work in progress.

Richard: We like to say that the progress never stops. There's constant rehabilitation your whole life, no matter how long you've had the cochlear implant, so that's understandable. Let me ask you about music. Does he enjoy music?

Michelle M. Wagner: He loves music. In fifth grade, he played the bongos for a school show. He likes happy music. He loves listening to The Chipmunks and has been to concerts with me. I don't know if you know who Michael Franti is, but he's very happy, upbeat music, and Mickey was right there in front of the stage. And the famous singer even gave my son his drum stick, and he loves music, loves it.

Richard: That's fantastic. I love that. That's great. I just must ask you one more question. As a parent, I want you to speak out to other parents who found out their children has a severe hearing loss. What advice would you give them? And I'm going to give you the floor to say anything you want.

Michelle M. Wagner: Embrace it, take every step in stride, and if you are secure in handling it and open to new ideas and willing to use every resource and do the work yourself, your child will be very successful, but the child has to feel safe. And there are resources for parents. There are parent groups where you can talk to, and that's the right place to let out your frustrations, and intimidation, or sadness, and utilize them. And talk openly with your family and friends. It's not something to hide for sure. It's an opportunity to educate. And every task is different. Every road is different. And I know because of certain challenges we overcame together, that he's happy and he's where he is today because-

Richard: That's fantastic. I appreciate your time. Your message will get out there. You've played it forward for hundreds. You have no clue who you're going to reach, so I really do appreciate your telling me the story.

Michelle M. Wagner: Thank you, Richard,

CHAPTER 16 SARAH SIMMONS TRULL

DISCOVERING YOUR CHILD IS DEAF. LESSONS FROM PARENTS ON THE COCHLEAR IMPLANT JOURNEY.

Finding out your child has a hearing loss can create a sense of total panic. What did we do wrong? How did we miss it? But after the panic subsides, the next question is, how do we deal with the situation? My parents must have gone through the same scenario, but they are no longer around for me to interview them. Fortunately, Sarah Simmons Trull agreed to talk about her and her husband's experience when they discovered their two year old son had a severe hearing loss. This interview gives us the opportunity to understand the hearing loss from the parents' point of view and how Sarah and her husband were able to deal with it.

Sarah Simmons Trull: My name is Sarah Trull, I am in Dallas, Texas, and it is February 12th, 2021

Richard: Tell me a little bit about your child's hearing loss, how you discovered it. How old was your child at the time?

Sarah Simmons Trull: He was late diagnosed when we found out. He was two and a half. We knew that there was something going on because he had a few words at one and then lost them, wasn't talking anymore, and so we had a sedated ABR that he had bilateral loss. One ear was worse than the other, and we went through genetics and found out that he has Pendred syndrome. My husband and I both carry the recessive gene, so we had no family history of hearing loss at all, and really no idea what to do initially and how to help him, so it was a journey for sure.

Richard: This is very important. What did you notice about his behavior at the time that made you suspicious? Was there a day, a moment, something happened?

Sarah Simmons Trull: He was so observant to visual stimulus that he would respond to our voices, we thought, but we didn't find out until he was in a preschool or a mother's day out program, and they said, "Do you think that he is not hearing well?" Later, we found out, too, with Pendred, he had enlarged vestibular aqueducts and a slight Mondini, so it can fluctuate, hearing can fluctuate. It's also progressive. I think, just him not talking was really our red flag.

Richard: You received the hint from the preschool. You and your husband, what were the first reaction you had?

Sarah Simmons Trull: We wanted to find out why he wasn't meeting those speech and language milestones. When it was finally diagnosed, I think I was relieved because I knew, "Okay, now we kind of know what to do as far as we can start helping him. We know the cause of why he's not talking, why he isn't progressing," but my husband was devastated.

Richard: Your husband. What about you?

Sarah Simmons Trull: I was actually glad to know what it was, to know like, "Oh, this is the cause, so now we can start working on other things to help him."

Richard: What steps did you take at that point to help him?

Sarah Simmons Trull: Everything was new to us, and I think, now even working as a professional, because I actually went back to school after going on this journey with him, I'm a speech pathologist now. I think it's really hard to navigate, initially. It's a whole new world. There's all this language that you don't really understand, a lot of misinformation, a lot of really strong opinions about communication options. It's just really hard to navigate as a parent.

Richard: Did you decide to get a cochlear implant at the time or were you looking for other options? How did you make a decision?

Sarah Simmons Trull: We weren't sure. He had hearing aids a little bit, but he wasn't really benefiting from them due to his degree of hearing loss. We wanted to make the right decision and it's hard, when you have a small child, to put them through surgery. But I think my husband and I both agreed that it was the best option for him.

Richard: Some parents, I see it on social media, when they discover the child is a candidate for a cochlear implant, a lot of discussion comes out, "Well, you shouldn't be making the decision for your child." There's a lot of controversy in that area. Tell me how you felt about that.

Sarah Simmons Trull: I saw some of that and I wanted to learn more about why that was said. But I think, for me, from looking at the research, we don't get that choice. There's a critical window for him. Children who are prelingually deaf, there's a window for auditory development and language development. Even if I wanted to give him that choice, which wasn't really an option. I guess, for us, we thought we're going to provide him with this, and if one day he chooses he doesn't want to hear, that's fine. He can have that choice and take them off. He doesn't hear when he takes them off, he doesn't hear anything, so I guess it's something where he could make that choice later. But if he wanted to get an implant later and he didn't have language, he wouldn't be able to do that.

Richard: That does make sense. I'll let the controversy roll on elsewhere, but I wanted to know your side of it.

Richard: He was two and a half when you found out he had a problem. How old was he when he got the cochlear implant?

Sarah Simmons Trull: I was pregnant with my second child, so we wanted to hurry it up, the process, so we got him scheduled sooner, so he got it when he was two years nine months, is when he had his surgery.

Richard: Very young. Did he do bilateral or single at the time?

Sarah Simmons Trull: Bilateral.

Richard: He did bilateral. The operation was done in Dallas, or where were you having it done?

Sarah Simmons Trull: It was in Dallas at Children's Medical Center with Dr. Brian Isaacson through the Callier Cochlear Implant program.

Sarah Simmons Trull: It was super hard to put your child through surgery, it's a hard decision, but he did so well. He was up and trying to play right as we left. It really wasn't bad. It wasn't bad.

Richard: I'd like to take you back one step. You met with the surgeon before surgery. What were the questions you asked and how did you feel about the answers you were getting?

Sarah Simmons Trull: I think one thing that I had read that was a concern is, because he did have a little bit of residual hearing, is if he would still have that. There is a lot of misinformation out there, unfortunately. I think I was reading a book one time and it said it's a one-shot, so if it doesn't work the first time you can't redo the surgery, which is not true, and things like that and just different outcomes. I did ask him about that. We didn't know which one to choose. There were three companies at the time. I think there are still three companies, cochlear implant manufacturers. That was a huge decision. We wanted to make the right decision for that, too, but I think, because of my son's anatomy, he was only able to choose from two different companies.

Richard: Which one did he choose?

Sarah Simmons Trull: Cochlear.

Richard: Now, tell me about surgery day. You took him to the hospital that day, your heart is in your mouth, and he came out of surgery and then what?

Sarah Simmons Trull: It was hard. It was great because he went, at the time, too, we actually transitioned him to a deaf preschool for kiddos who are looking at cochlear implants, are thinking about wanting to develop oral language. His teacher came by his speech therapist came by, so that was nice. We had a great community already being in that world such a short time. I think we were excited but scared.

Richard: That's natural. Now, did he continue with the deaf school or is he just didn't know?

Sarah Simmons Trull: He did for a few months, but then we decided to put him in a mainstream kindergarten classroom, and now he's 10 and he's in fourth grade and mainstreamed fully.

Richard: Fully mainstream. And he's happy?

Sarah Simmons Trull: He is. Yeah. There are still some challenges for him with listening. The teacher wears an FM so he can hear better, but he's such a smart kiddo. He advocates for himself in the classroom, which is great.

Richard: Can you talk about some of the challenges, more of the challenges he had? I'm sure people would like to know more about that.

Sarah Simmons Trull: Absolutely. I think the main thing for a kiddo that's hearing impaired and who hears with cochlear implants, the hearing is different than the way a hearing person hears. Being able to hear in a noisy classroom with... Kids are loud, so it's very noisy and a lot of classrooms are not set up acoustically to make the environment where kids can hear instruction. We asked our school district to provide an FM system to where the teacher wears a mic that goes directly into his processor so he can hear the teacher as if she was standing next to him. That was really a big thing for us.

Sarah Simmons Trull: Also, vocabulary is hard for him because he must have more exposure to it than a typical hearing kid. He misses certain things sometimes just from not being able to hear people talking over here or things that are incidental learning opportunities, I guess, also when he was younger. But he does a great job of asking questions and, if there is a communication breakdown, trying to repair that, even with him, because his speech has come a long way, but sometimes we have to remind him, "Oh, can you tell me again or can you say it a different way?" Or "That wasn't clear, can you repeat that?" And he does those things.

Richard: I want to get back to speech therapy in a second, but I want to also ask you, because I mentor people in 24 time zones, and there are so many different cultural aspects about getting a cochlear implant that some parents won't do it because they're afraid their child is going to stand out. In fact, I mentored one family in Ireland where the husband needed the CI, and he didn't want to do it because his child would be bullied that the father had it. My question to you is, culturally, what's going on? Do the children accept it? Does he have to fend for himself? Is he bullied? What goes on at that point?

Sarah Simmons Trull: When he was young, kids would notice it, and kids are cruel sometimes and they just say whatever, they don't have a filter. When kids would point it out, I would say, "Oh, isn't that cool? That helps him hear." And kind of explain it to the other kids. It's cool because I didn't realize that I was modeling that for him, but I've heard him tell other kids, "Yeah, God gave me this implant so that I could hear." He was just like, "Yeah, this is so I can hear." Like I wear my glasses so I can see.

Sarah Simmons Trull: I think his perspective of it is great, and so other kids notice that, too. It's not a big deal to him. That's just something that may be different than the way other kids hear, but it's not a big issue. He's very charismatic and has such a great personality, I think. He does really well. Because we worried about that for sure, about bullying. When a child has something that's different from other kids, you worry that, "Oh, that could be a target." But I think I've been really impressed with the way he's handled that.

Richard: I now want to go to speech therapy because that's your vocation. Tell me a little bit about did he need speech therapy once he got hearing? Tell me what happened at that point?

Sarah Simmons Trull: He was late diagnosed, didn't start talking until he was four and a half, and we did auditory verbal approach. We had a great speech therapist that really helped him develop listening skills first before speech. I think that's really helped him now just doing that oral rehab. But he still is in speech at school. I work with him some at home, too. He'll probably need that for a while. I think if he would have been identified earlier, I wonder if he wouldn't have needed that as much, just because he would have had those early auditory experiences.

Richard: It is water under the bridge now. We understand that. But one of the things I'm trying to make parents aware of, the earlier the better, if they're going to get speech properly, that's fine. I think you've covered a lot, but I know you probably have something you'd like to share with parents who are in the same situation you're in with your son. Would you like to tell us a little bit more?

Sarah Simmons Trull: I think what you said is spot on. The earlier, the better. Even as a clinician, as a speech pathologist, I have a couple of kiddos on my caseload and I used to mentor for Cochlear Americas, too. Parents would feel pressure. I want to make the right decision and there's this sense of urgency. Then I've heard other professionals say, "Oh, take your time. You don't have to make a decision today." But knowing what I know now as a parent and a professional, I would say, as soon as you can do it, if it's the right option for you and your family, go ahead and do it. You can't get that time back.

Sarah Simmons Trull: The brain is set up to receive that auditory information because of the high plasticity. You can't get those years back. In retrospect, if we would've known, we would have not hesitated. At the time, it was a very hard decision, but now it was the best decision that I think we could have made for him or have ever made for him. It's been such a blessing to him and his life, thinking about how creative he is, even with the way he communicates with friends and for him to not have that ability to communicate with peers, we're so thankful that we were given the right information for us as a family and had those opportunities to get the cochlear implant and pursue it.

Richard: I think that perspective is going to be extremely important for people who come on to the website for the first time looking for information, because it's so confusing and it's such a major decision to make. I really do appreciate your sharing this with us. I want to thank you so much for your time today.

Sarah Simmons Trull:

Thank you so much. Thank you for having me.

Chapter 17 Chery Edwards Part 1

Struggled with Meniere's Disease and Deafness. How Chery Got Her Life Back. Pre-Op Interview

Meniere's disease is insidious. It not only causes severe vestibular balance issues, but it also often leaves its victims deaf in one ear or both.

Chery Edwards was such a victim when she was hit with Meniere's 20 years ago. Her vestibular issues caused bouts of vertigo which caused her to give up driving. She could never predict when it would strike and cause her to lose control of her car.

It also left her deaf in one ear.

Although Chery is among one of the most positive personalities I have met, she was also resigned to her fate. That was until she recently saw a YouTube video with Dr. Herb Silverstein, who described a possible solution to the symptoms of Meniere's. Traveling from Denver to Sarasota, she had a consultation at the Silverstein Institute. She will receive a Labyrinthectomy to remove her middle ear and resolve the vertigo issues and simultaneously receive a cochlear implant to bring back her hearing with a Cochlear Nucleus 7.

Chery describes her struggles with Meniere's and her upcoming operation which will be performed by Dr. Jack Wazen at Silverstein.

This interview is in two parts, the pre-op, and the post activation.

Richard: Do you want to tell me a little bit about your hearing loss? When did you get Meniere's disease or when did you start to lose your hearing?

Chery Edwards: I had my first Meniere's attack when I was about 36, 37 years old. I was diagnosed at 37 and that was about 20 years ago. It was about 1999.

Richard: You told me before, you haven't been able to drive a car since then.

Chery Edwards: That was progressive. Meniere's disease is typically progressive. The attacks come and go and when they hit you, the fullness in the ear, the vertigo, dizziness, nausea, and vomiting, all that stuff hit you. And then it usually takes several hours of sleeping afterwards to kind of recuperate from the attack. And as you have more and more attacks, your hearing is slowly decreased until eventually you're deaf. It took me about, oh, just under five years to go deaf.

Richard: Your deafness is on one side?

Chery Edwards: It's on the one side. It's on left. Yes.

Richard: Five years of progressive loss, too.

Chery Edwards: Yeah. Yeah. That's exactly how it goes. And then I'll never forget the time I went in, and they did a hearing test, and I asked the doctor, I said, "Do you think it's going to come back this time?" And he said, "No." He said, "Your hearing is gone, and it will never come back." He was right. It never did.

Richard: What did you feel that day when he told you that?

Chery Edwards: Well, of course, I wasn't happy about it. I'm a tough person when it comes to strengths, so I just accepted that I was going to have to live with just the hearing in one ear. Probably the largest fear that I've ever had was that I would develop bilateral Meniere's disease and then go completely deaf in both ears.

Richard: Did you ever meet anybody who with bilateral Meniere's?

Chery Edwards: I have met people on Facebook, but never in person that are bilateral. Yep.

Richard: At this point, they don't think it's going to spread to the other side.

Chery Edwards: They don't think so. It's not typical for someone that has had Meniere's disease for as long as I have, but it does happen. The most recent attack that I had really did scare me because it was the worst one I've ever had. It lasted for about 16, 17 hours.

Richard: Talk to me a little bit about what that felt like at that time.

Chery Edwards: I woke up in the morning and the room was spinning so much so that I couldn't get out of bed. That's the only way you can describe it. You can't walk, you can't get up. You can't even really roll over in bed because you don't know which way is up.

Richard: Is there a nausea involved in it or not?

Chery Edwards: Yes, very much so. Yeah. There's violent throwing up that goes with it. This attack, the symptoms were not any longer just in my left side. I had the fullness in the ear and the strong tinnitus was in my good ear this time, and so that really scared me and that's how I've ended up finding the Silverstein Institute here in Florida because I was doing research to try and figure out what I could do.

Richard: You're visiting here from Denver because you've heard that Silverstein is the best Institute dealing with Meniere's.

Chery Edwards: That's true, yes.

Richard: Where did you find out about him?

Chery Edwards: I just found a YouTube video. I was researching and researching, and I found a video that he was interviewed, and it's the first time I had ever heard a doctor say, Meniere's patients are just told that they must live with it and there's nothing that can be done for them. That is not true. There are things that we can do. And when I heard him say that I was like, "Where is this man? I have to go find him." So, that's how I found the Silverstein Institute.

Richard: It's all about the education. It's all about finding out what the truth is of your disease [inaudible 00:06:06].

Chery Edwards: Absolutely.

New Speaker: Absolutely. There are very, very few physicians that are high level specialists in Meniere's disease. They're hard to find.

Richard: You were very lucky to find them.

Chery Edwards: I was absolutely.

Richard: Since this happened about 20 years ago when you had your first attack, am I right?

Chery Edwards: Mm-hmm (affirmative). Yep.

Richard: What happened to your career, your family? What was going on at that time?

Chery Edwards: Well, like I said, Meniere's is progressive and different patients have different triggers. My triggers for attacks and that caused it to get worse in general are fatigue, so lack of sleep and dehydration if I don't drink enough water and stress. I was married to an abusive husband for 27 years. I had six children and ran a mortgage company, so my stress level was extreme. I'm assuming that's why I got it to begin with.

Chery Edwards: I continued to manage that life until it was about the time that, or maybe a couple of years before I left my ex, so it would have been about 2009 that this happened. I'd be sitting at my desk working with someone or taking a loan application, and suddenly have an attack, like a drop attack that was just instant, and I couldn't finish, I couldn't function.

Chery Edwards: When that happened. I quit working and then went into applying for social security disability and all of that. I've been on SSDI for about eight years now.

Richard: I want to ask you about the relationship with your husband. Did he leave because of the disease, because of what you're going through or was that something separate?

Chery Edwards: No. I left him. His abuse was primarily emotional and psychological.

Richard: Okay. That's fine.

Chery Edwards: Because he wasn't hitting me, I didn't recognize that I was being abused or that my children were. I knew there was a problem, but it was like I couldn't put my finger on why. I always thought it was my fault, which is very typical. I've learned a lot about abuse and how it all functions since then, but when I realized that's what I was experiencing, I just said, "I'm leaving. I'm not going to stay in this." And I did.

Richard: I appreciate your telling me that because a lot of what we talk about in the Hearing Loss Association is the relationship issues with hearing loss with their spouse or significant other, and that's why I was asking you if your hearing had something to do with that relationship.

Chery Edwards: Yeah. Well, it did in that I truly believe that the stress that he caused by abusing me and of course the children, I was his primary target, but I believe that that stress was probably the reason. In fact, I have an aunt that says, "It's so interesting that he abused you with words and it was your hearing that went. It's almost like your body knew that's what needed to go."

Richard: Okay, that makes sense. Your career changed. You couldn't use the phone anymore. You can use the phone-

Chery Edwards: I can use the phone because I do have perfect hearing in my right ear to this day. I can use a phone. It wasn't the phone that was a problem for me. It was the attacks at the time. The one thing with the phone that's true, if you have any other people that have single-sided deafness like me, you can't talk on the phone and understand anything else that's going on around you. You know how a lot of times you'll be talking on the phone, and somebody will talk to you thinking you can hear both people? It's like, sorry, that's not happening.

Richard: You know, that's very interesting because a lot of people with normal hearing can't multi-task either if they're on the phone. They can't understand what anybody is saying, so it's not necessarily the hearing issue in this case.

Chery Edwards: That's true.

Richard: You had support from your family?

Chery Edwards: My kids have been incredibly supportive. Yes. I've been very, very fortunate. That makes me emotional when I think about it.
Richard: That's okay.

Chery Edwards: They have been there for me in ways. Right now, I have an elderly mother that has Alzheimer's. I'm her caregiver. My daughter is taking time off work to take care of her grandmother so that I can be down here and do this. I'm very, very blessed to have amazing kids. Yeah.

Richard: You know you have perfect hearing on one side so that when you're taking care of your mother you have full access to what anybody's telling you, which-

Chery Edwards: Well, that is one of the reasons why I really feel strongly about needing a CI. There's a couple of things. One, I have zero directional hearing, so if there is a sound that happens that I need to know what's going on, it is completely impossible for me to tell you where the sound is coming from. That's one thing.

Chery Edwards: I very often sleep on my good ear, it's easier to go to sleep that way. I go to sleep on my good ear. If something happened with mom while I was sleeping, there's no way I would know.

Richard: Do you still have tinnitus from the...?

Chery Edwards: I have severe tinnitus in my left ear. I'm profoundly deaf in my left ear and just since this last attack in June, I have tinnitus in my good ear now. Tinnitus and fullness in the ear that comes and goes. The tinnitus is worse, but yes, so these are the reasons I'm concerned about possibly going bilateral with them in years.

Richard: Even if you have an operation and you get a cochlear implant on your deaf side, you're going to take it off at night and you're still going to be deaf on that side.

Chery Edwards: I've thought of that, yes, and that sort of is what it is. One of the questions that I've had is can I leave it on? And if that side is up when I'm sleeping on my good ear, can I leave it on? That's one of the questions that I had for you.

Richard: That's going to be a great question to ask because generally they tell you not to wear a cochlear implant at night so that your brain gets some rest.

Chery Edwards: Okay.

Richard: But I'm not a doctor, I'm not a surgeon. It's another side of the coin without going-

Chery Edwards: Well, we'll ask Dr. Wazen.

217

Richard: We'll get there when you get there.

Chery Edwards: Yeah, yeah.

Richard: Your expectations are?

Chery Edwards: Well, I am having a labyrinthectomy done on the 19th of November, so that's in about three weeks. And that I'm really excited about because when they take that out, the labyrinth is the balance center of the inner ear in the affected ear. When they take that out, it stops the vertigo in its tracks. For the first time in 20 years, I'll be able to drive. I won't have attacks anymore.

Richard: Why couldn't they have removed that long ago?

Chery Edwards: They could have if I had known about it, but I didn't. I never ran into a doctor that even told me about it. When I heard Dr. Silverstein say he could do something for me, I was just like, "Wherever I have to go, whatever I have to do, we're going to get this figured out."

Richard: It is very common in the sense that most doctors, general practitioners, and people who are not in the ENT side of the medicine, they're totally ignorant about cochlear implants.

Chery Edwards: Yes. Even ENTs. I saw an ENT, and of course, I won't mention her name, but I saw an ENT before I came down here and all she did was give me a diuretic that also lowers your blood pressure. I do not have high blood pressure. It caused me to pass out dead cold on the floor from that medication. It was like, clearly this is a specialist, it was an ENT, but she does not have a clue about Meniere's disease.

Richard: It's always true. We struggle till we find the right doctor, no matter what our symptoms are.

Chery Edwards: Yes, yes. That's very, very true for Meniere's patients. It really is. Just like you're on a Facebook for a cochlear implant, I'm on another one that's for Meniere's patients, and it's just daily that there's posts on there where people can't find a doctor that can really help them. Yeah.

Richard: Oh, my gosh.

Chery Edwards: I'm very blessed and grateful. Very grateful.

Richard: We call our guardian angels watching after us to find the right doctor.

Chery Edwards: Yes, exactly. Really, really, grateful. Yeah.

Richard: Let me ask you a little bit more about the operation. As you understand it, they're going to be removing the balance center.

Chery Edwards: The labyrinth. Yeah.

Richard: Simultaneously, they're going to be inserting a cochlear implant... correct?

Chery Edwards: That's I'm here for right now is to do the cochlear implant evaluation and we are shooting for approval with the insurance company, which Dr. Wazen thinks that we can get done so that when he goes into the labyrinthectomy he can also put the cochlear implant in at the same time. That's the goal.

Richard: This is a brand-new aspect of cochlear implants the singlesided deafness.

Chery Edwards: Yes.

Richard: Until recently, doctors who were doing it were doing it outside the prescribed regulations because single-sided deafness in cochlear implants, insurance companies don't want to pay for it. Medicare wouldn't pay for it. It's just a growing issue right now.

Chery Edwards: Well, there's good reason for it. For example, like I said, I have six children. They all have significant others. Now, they're older and grown and out of the house. Just a month or so ago, I went to a restaurant with all my kids and my new husband for dinner with a family. Right? I may as well have been completely deaf. I could not hear anything that anyone had to say.

Chery Edwards: So that is a reality for people that are single-sided deaf, is that there's all kinds of little things that you don't expect, and I'm sure insurance companies that make these decisions wouldn't know. I have written a letter to them to be submitted with my CI evaluation just about quality of life. So that entire time I sat there for an hour. I enjoyed watching my family laugh and have a good time, but I was not part of it.

Richard: But you were in isolation.

Chery Edwards: I was completely isolated. I would drive down the road with my husband and he tries to talk to me. My deafness is in the ear that's towards the driver's seat. I can't hear him when he talks to me. He must speak up loudly and I have to turn and look right at him to be able to hear him.

Richard: I had to lip read for 35 years while I was driving.

Chery Edwards: I cannot imagine that. Your story is so incredible to me. It really, really is.

Richard: You're hoping to get that aspect?

Chery Edwards: Oh, absolutely. And the directional hearing, able to hear where things are coming from, able to drive again. The labyrinthectomy is going to give me that ability. I'm really excited about that. But the hearing piece for me is there's so much that I've missed, and I know that. My family surprised me with... I have a son that was gone to Germany with the military for three years and I hadn't seen him in three years. And they surprised me by having him be in my house when I got home. I made a trip to Texas and came back and walked in the house and there he was.

Chery Edwards: One of my other sons said something early, would have ruined the surprise, right beside me. But he was on my deaf side, so I completely missed it. In that case, it was a good thing because the surprise was amazing. But how many-

Richard: Your son might have surprised you didn't react when he-
Chery Edwards: No, no. He knew.

Richard: But you didn't react when he said.

Chery Edwards: It was one of those things where I heard somebody on this side say, "She didn't hear you," and I turned to look and he just kind of walked off and I was like, "oh, well I guess it wasn't..." You know, whatever. And later I found out that was-

Richard: Does your family ever use the expression when you couldn't hear something, oh, that's not important or I'll tell you later?

Chery Edwards: Oh, all the time. All the time.

Richard: How does that make you feel?

Chery Edwards: Oh, it just frustrates me. I'm outspoken now.

Richard: Let's talk about it.

Chery Edwards: I didn't use to be.

Richard: Let's talk about that for a bit. The "Never mind."

Chery Edwards: I didn't used to mind. Yeah. It's okay.se to be, but now I'm just like, "Don't do that to me. If you spoke something, it was because you intended for me to hear it. If I didn't hear you, I'll turn around so that I can hear you, but don't just go, 'Oh, never mind. It doesn't matter.'

If it didn't matter, you wouldn't have said it in the first place."

Richard: Exactly right.

Chery Edwards: So, I'm open about it. But yes, it happens all the time.

Richard: We talk about that all the time at the hearing loss association meetings. It's the most painful when somebody says, "Oh, it doesn't matter."

Chery Edwards:

Richard:

Chery Edwards: It's almost like discounting that you are in the room when they say that. That's how it feels. The other thing, and this is my bad, I'm not good at saying what enough. I will assume that I understood what they said, and I'll respond and they're like, "No." I did that to [Chavez 00:00:19:02] just... Was it yesterday? Yeah.

Richard: You do know you'll continue lip reading after you get this anyway.

Chery Edwards: I hadn't thought of that.

Richard: You will. It still becomes a very natural part of your life to be lip reading them. I can understand somebody if I'm not watching them, but if I'm talking to somebody-

Chery Edwards: You're still doing it.

Richard: You still lip read.

Chery Edwards: Well, I naturally, without thinking of it now, always turn my good ear side to whatever. If I'm sitting down anywhere- Richard: That [inaudible 00:19:30].

Chery Edwards: I want to turn that way so that I can be a part of what's going on.

Richard: You're going to hopefully have the operation. You're still in the stage of evaluation, and if they go ahead, you'll come back to the operation and you'll stay for how long?

Chery Edwards: The operation will be on the 19th of November, which is in about three weeks, and then I'll stay here in Florida for two weeks and then fly back. Dr. Wazen did give me permission to fly two weeks after, so go back to Denver.

Richard: Will you be activated here or back in Denver?

Chery Edwards: I don't know the answer to that question.

Richard: We will find out.

Chery Edwards: Yeah, yeah.

Richard: That's fine. That's okay. That's fine.

Chery Edwards: From what I understand, a major part of Cochlear is in Denver so we may be able to get me activated up there.

Richard: You understand what I'm trying to do here is part one of a two-part interview.

Chery Edwards: Yes, I do.

Richard: We'll do another interview by Skype. When you get back and you're activated, and we can talk about the changes then.

Chery Edwards: Sure.

Richard: Because I want to know how you're feeling now, what you're looking for. Do you have any hobbies that depend on your hearing or...?

Chery Edwards: My dad was a music teacher, and I grew up with music all around me. Always loved it, had a very powerful singing voice as a younger person and did a lot of singing through school, a lot of solo work and that kind of thing. I can't do that anymore because my hearing is... You would think that having hearing in one ear would be good enough to still be able to hear tones and stuff, and it is sometimes, but it's not consistent enough for me to rely on it.

Richard: That's going to be very interesting to follow up on because the cochlear implant, music, it's a very personal topic and I'm looking forward to seeing if you get your voice back.

Chery Edwards: It would mean the world to me to be able to sing again. Yes. That's in the letter that I put together for... Hopefully the insurance...

Richard: I wish I have the letter.

Chery Edwards: I'll get it to you. I can email it to you.

Richard: If you send me letter, I'll read it out.

Chery Edwards: Sure.

Richard: And add it to this before we post it.

Chery Edwards: Absolutely.

Richard: I would love to see that.

Chery Edwards: I'm happy to do that.

Richard: If this works, Lord willing, this works, what are your goals for the future when you have the implant?

Chery Edwards: I want to get off social security disability. I want to work again. I want to drive again. I'm going to have my life back by the grace of God.

Richard: They're all doable. Everything you said is doable.

Chery Edwards: Absolutely. I think it is. It's kind of surreal. It's like, I'm going to have my life back.

Richard: I know you're tearing up with the thought, but that's fine.

Chery Edwards: Yeah.

Richard: We all walked in your moccasins, but you have slightly different ones.

Chery Edwards: I do. I do. And I have a real passion for helping people that are in my situation. Because there's so many circumstances where people look at you and they think you're fine and- Richard: It's an invisible disability.

Chery Edwards: It is invisible and it's difficult unless a person has been there with you when you have an attack or has been deaf, so they live with that kind of issue. They don't really understand. It gives me a real passion to reach out to people that are struggling with what I'm struggling with, especially on the other side, after being able to, like I said, Lord willing, being able to drive again and all of those things, and just reach out to people and say, "Hey, there's hope." You don't have to live for 20 years like I did with this.

Richard: Now that's a fantastic attitude. That's what I love to hear. As far as choosing which company you're going with, you haven't a made decision yet. You're doing that at some point with Dr. Wazen and Dr. Silverstein, I'm sure.

Chery Edwards: Yeah, I'll probably go with Cochlear. I've already been in contact with their rep, and I just adore her. She's amazing. I can't imagine looking elsewhere, but that's just my personal experience.

Richard: Anything you would like to add for people who are potential candidates who might be sitting on the fence?

Chery Edwards: I understand the fear. I think for the same reasons that a lot of people are afraid, but to me it's like life is short just get it done so that you can enjoy it to the fullest. We're only here for so long and we never know exactly how long that's going to be, so don't hold yourself back. That's how I feel about it. I'm jumping in with both feet, man, double surgery in the same day.

Richard: All right. I hope you're up dancing in the aisles by [inaudible 00:23:52].

Chery Edwards: Yes. Yeah.

Richard: All right. Well, Chery, I thank you so much for your time.

Chery Edwards: Oh, thank you.

Richard: I really appreciate your insights and I'm sure other people who are candidates for cochlear implants are going to get quite a bit from this. Thank you so much.

Chery Edwards: Well, thank you, Richard. I really, really appreciate what you're doing. You empower people and that's admirable. I really appreciate that.

Richard: Thank you so much.

CHAPTER 18 CHERY EDWARDS PART 2

HOW CHERY GOT HER GROOVE BACK. PART 2 AFTER SURGERY

This is Part 2 of the interview with Chery Edwards. It is almost two months post-operation. She flew from Denver, Colorado to Sarasota, Florida to receive a labyrinthectomy and be simultaneously implanted with a cochlear implant by Dr. Jack Wazen at the Silverstein Institute.

Chery returned home after two weeks recovery for the labyrinthectomy. She was activated in Colorado and has had three MAP sessions with her audiologist after receiving a Cochlear Nucleus 7.

This was the ideal opportunity to catch up with her while her reactions to the experience are still fresh and to talk about her recovery, rehab and how she is experiencing the issues of her Meniere's as well as hearing. Her insights about music are also invaluable.

Chery has a remarkable and inspiring story.

Richard: Good morning.

Chery Edwards: Good morning.

Richard: We're talking with Chery Edward this morning and part two of our original interview. And Chery, you had surgery on November 19th,

2020. I don't have the date when you were activated. Could you describe the recovery from your surgery?

Chery Edwards: Well, of course, as you know, I had a labyrinthectomy as well as the cochlear implant done and recovery from the labyrinthectomy was tough, especially the first two, three days. Just the vertigo and balance issues. That's normal and it gets better as you work hard at your vestibular exercises; it gets better over the weeks. Well, I was activated on December 11th to answer your question about that, but I would say now, I'm coming up on two months. On the 19th, it'll be two months since surgery and my balance is probably about 85, 90% consistently. The exercises that they have me doing that are intense are the hard ones, but I'll get there.

Richard: So, the question is, what kind of exercises...? How many hours a day do you have to do them? Is it every day or...?

Chery Edwards: It is every day. I usually do them between an hour and a half and two hours a day. I break them up in half hour slots and they consist of different ways of moving your eyes, different ways, whether you're standing or sitting, they have a balance. It's like a cushion that they have you stand on when you're doing some of these harder ones. And what it does is, it challenges your balance so that your brain can learn how to balance with just one labyrinth.

Richard: But every day it's a little bit better or is it like a plateau [inaudible 00:03:51]?

Chery Edwards: It would make more sense to measure it like from week to week as opposed to day to day, because day to day, a lot of times you can't tell the difference, but when you look back a week or more, you can tell.

Richard: That's on your balance side. What about activation day? When you had the implant activated? What was that like?

Chery Edwards: That was exciting. Sort of weird. Everything was incredibly loud, so that took some getting used to. It was good that I had some practice with having tinnitus for a long time. I wore it anyway, even though everything was loud. My audiologist said I had a great activation. I was able to understand some words. She sounded mechanical, but I was able to understand some words through activation, which I understand I'm very, very blessed. I think it's a [crosstalk 00:04:46].

Richard: Absolutely. And ever since activation day your hearing's gotten better?

Chery Edwards: Yeah. I've just been working hard on practicing and listening, and I'm convinced that that makes a huge difference.

Richard: Can you describe what you're doing for listening practice? People want to know that.

Chery Edwards: Mostly what I do is I'll get an audio book on my phone and then I'll order the hard copy and I read while I'm listening, so that's been helpful. When I'm running around the house doing chores or whatever, I do a lot of just streaming directly to the CI. I walk on the treadmill at the same time streaming to my CI with the TV streamer and the close captions off. I usually do that for about an hour, to an hour and a half every day. So those are all things that really help. And yesterday I just got some new Bose headphones and I'm absolutely in love.

Richard: Tell us about the Bose headphones. What happens?

Chery Edwards: Well, because I am fortunate enough to only be deaf on one side, my good ear hears the full sound, like a natural ear would and I think it's going to help to train my CI because for the first time in 15 years I now have stereo sound. I can't even put it into words how amazing that is. It's so awesome.

Richard: What did you play first when you put the stereo sound on?

What were you listening to?

Chery Edwards: Well, Karen Carpenter is one of my favorite old...

from teenage years. Mostly jazz. I love jazz and old seventies stuff. The mellow seventies stuff.

Richard: I found jazz easiest to recover, to use for rehabilitation too because anything with swing with a lot of brass just seems to be easier.

Chery Edwards: Yeah, I've noticed that with jazz too. It's good to hear you say that because I'll stream it more. I mean, these poor headphones are going to get used a lot.

Richard: Same thing, same thing. I went to Best Buy, I tried on every single pair of headsets before I decided on one. How did you decide on the Bose?

Chery Edwards: Well, I know Bose because we have a Bose stereo system and stuff. I've always loved them. I know they're expensive, but they're worth it, and I looked at the size of the inside of the earpiece that covers your ear, and I picked the one that's not the highest level. It's the next to the highest level because it had the largest opening and I wanted to make sure I covered the microphones well.

Richard: I did the same thing.

Chery Edwards: Did you?

Richard: That's good. Absolutely, the same time. Tell me a little bit about speech. How's that coming along?

Chery Edwards: Speech recognition, oh my God. I've been fortunate to have the activation and then three mappings since activation. This last one, she tested me with sentences, and I got 96% speech recognition. I was absolutely blown away and it is still echo-y. It still sounds loud, and it echoes. That's the best way, a bit muffled maybe. But if I focus and pay attention, that's the level at which... I mean, to be that way a month after activation... I'm very aware that a lot of people don't get to have these kinds of results right away. And I'm just humbled and grateful beyond measure.

Richard: May I ask you again, I want to go back to the headset because you do have natural hearing in one ear and the CI and the other.

Chery Edwards: That's correct.

Richard: So, tell me a little bit about how that sounds.

Chery Edwards: Well, of course in my good ear, it sounds incredibly gorgeous through Bose headphones. I always turn the app on to the music setting and I would say tinny is one of the words I would use to describe it. Also, I don't hear pitch nearly as well, so when I'm using the Bose headphones, I find myself just closing my eyes and trying to tell my brain, this is the pitch, this is where we're at, because I can hear it clearly with my good ear. I'm very blessed.

Richard: So, music's coming back?

Chery Edwards: It is. I was telling my husband last night, I really feel like I'm getting music back, especially growing up with my dad as a music teacher and stuff. There are no words you can put to that, that say how meaningful that is. It's just incredible. And this is just the beginning.

Richard: Music is so important.

Chery Edwards: Yeah, it really is. Yeah.

Richard: You sent me a clip of you playing the flute. I was blown away. How long ago was it you played the flute?

Chery Edwards: Oh, probably 35 years. Yeah, so I'm incredibly rusty. Richard: It was beautiful. Beautiful piece, I was very...

Chery Edwards: Well, thank you. Kind of like riding a bike. I noticed with practicing yesterday. The first time it took me a little bit to go, Oh yeah. And then it just started to come back. I've got lots of practicing in my future though as well. And I want to do the same with the piano because from what I understand, to train your brain, it's kind of like speech and reading. If you speak it, you write it and you read it, you do all those things and you listen to it, it's part of how we learn to speak. Music is the same way. If you play it, you read it on the music and you're listening to it at the same time, it's supposed to help your brain catch on.

Richard: You're obviously doing a good job with it.

Chery Edwards: I feel so new at this still, but just beyond thrilled with my results.

Richard: Now, your balance is coming back a bit and you told us in your first interview you haven't driven in 20 years. Do you have plans to go back?

Chery Edwards: Well, on that interview I got off on another subject talking about CIs and I didn't answer that. I haven't driven in eight years. I've had Meniere's for 20 years. So, I am seriously looking forward to getting to the place where the vestibular therapist releases me and said, "Yep, you can go get your license." And I expect that to probably be in the next month or six weeks.

Richard: We'll want to be there for your driving test.

Chery Edwards: Yeah. Oh, no. I'm not looking forward to that, but we'll get it done.

Richard: That's great. This is fabulous. I'm so happy for you, the results were spectacular.

Chery Edwards: Oh, thank you.

Richard: Would you like to say anything to everybody out there who's on the fence at this point?

Chery Edwards: I think I said this in the first interview. Life is short. Just do it. Just jump in with both feet. Give it your all. When you don't feel like it, push yourself to do the practicing. Just do it because it enriches your life in a way that you can't even put into words. For me, the ability to be able to have directional hearing now, is just huge. So, when a sound comes, even though it might not sound like it does in my right ear yet, at least I know where it's coming from. And that's a huge deal with single-sided deaf people because the sound, you have no idea where it's coming from. So yeah, I would just encourage people to reach out to people like you and myself and others that would support them and just walk the journey.

Chery Edwards: To be honest, recovering from the labyrinthectomy was much more difficult by far than the CI. Much more difficult. So, if all you're doing is just the CI recovery, yes, its surgery, but man, my experience was that it was not difficult.

Richard: I'm glad you had it done. I'm glad you're making such tremendous progress. We're all very proud of you.

Chery Edwards: Oh, thanks Richard.

Richard: Just amazing. So, thank you so much.

Chery Edwards: I want to take a moment too, to say thank you for all that you do. You work so hard to empower people, encourage them so that they can join the world of hearing again, and it just means so much to so many. So, I want to take a moment to just say thank you for that.

Richard: You're more than welcome. I get great pleasure when I hear success stories.

CHAPTER 19 VINELL LACY

EXPERIENCES OF A COCHLEAR IMPLANT CANDIDATE STILL ON THE FENCE

Vinell Lacy has a profound hearing loss with a long period of decline. Eventually, her hearing loss became so severe she had to give up her career, which she loved, as a legal secretary. Her story is compelling and frightening at times. She relates her inability to contact 9-1-1 because she could not hear on a phone. She is qualified for cochlear implants the time of this interview, but she has delayed it for reasons that she talks about. She has not chosen the company she will use when she is ready. Like many cochlear implant candidates, the choice can be overwhelming. Her story presents the view of a qualified cochlear implant candidate and the issues she has confronted.

Richard: I would like to know a little bit about your hearing loss, when you lost it, when you noticed you had a hearing loss. Tell me a little bit about that.

Vinell Lacy: I noticed I had a hearing loss when I was about 36 years old. I was told by a couple people that I didn't say good morning to them because I had a job where I work one-on-one at the time for an eye doctor. Then I moved to places at that point, and I started having ringing in my ears very bad. I went to the doctor, and they did a hearing test, and they could not believe that my hearing was so bad. They recommended hearing aids at that point. I went to the first audiologist and got hearing aids and it really didn't help me very much.

Richard: When you got the hearing aid, what did you experience?

Vinell Lacy: I just heard a lot of garbles. It just wasn't clear, nothing was clear. I could hear better without them, and I couldn't hear on the phone at all. I had to take them off to barely be able to hear on the phone. So, then I went to a different audiologist that I had come to the Hearing Loss Association, and I met Flo Innis, and she said you need to go to a different doctor. I did. And he really tried to help. He set me up with nice phones in my office, I worked for an attorney at the time, and it just did not help a lot.

Richard: Talk about that. You were working for an attorney, which was a job I believe you loved very much, and you start to lose your hearing. What was happening at the time in terms of your job?

Vinell Lacy: Well, I started working for an attorney in 2002, and this was about 2006 that I kept experiencing problems with hearing. The attorney would answer a lot of the phone calls for me because I could not take them.

Richard: How'd you feel about that?

Vinell Lacy: It was terrible. It was just terrible. But I was lucky because I'd worked for him for 18 years all together and he would rather help me then lose me, I guess. At this point, the hearing was so bad that I couldn't hear his dictation. It was getting bad.

Richard: He called you in his office and tried dictate something to you, and can you describe a little bit what happened on those occasions.

Vinell Lacy: Well, at this point he's like, "You know, we're going to have to do something because this is taking up a lot of time for you." So I went to the other audiologist that Flo had recommended, and they had gotten me set up with the Com Pilot and all that which helped a lot at this point. I was barely able to cope at this point. We got the new phone and had everything set up, but still wasn't good enough to get by. This was around 2006. Well, my attorney passed away suddenly, had a heart attack right in front of me. At this point, I'm a legal secretary and I cannot continue to be a legal secretary because I cannot hear. I cannot answer the phone and a couple the attorneys called and asked, "Can you come and work for me now?" I turned them down without even telling them why.

Richard: That's very interesting. Why didn't you tell them?

Vinell Lacy: I just knew I couldn't do it. At this point I wasn't familiar with how to handle my hearing loss. I felt alone at this point. I just kind of withdrew and went into a plumbing company where I didn't have to answer the phone, I didn't have to deal with the public. I could have a one-on-one world.

Richard: And you're still there at this point.

Vinell Lacy: Yes. In 2009, I decided I would purchase the plumbing company and I would get my license and become a plumber, because I didn't have to hear everything.

Richard: Who deals with the public in your company? If you have a problem hearing, there must a way you're compensating by having somebody take the phone. Is there-

Vinell Lacy: Yes, and in my business, I have really a big disadvantage because as a small company with only my son and myself, he does the work in the fields, and I can't answer the phones. It's really put me into a real bad disadvantage of not being able to really work in my own company with just hearing aids.

Richard: Okay. If you have that disadvantage of the only other person being in the field, you can't answer the phones, what's the future hold for you?

Vinell Lacy: It's hard. It's very hard.

Richard: You must run three times harder to get the same thing done.
Vinell Lacy: Yes. Yes.

Richard: You have your audiologist since you've been here. What's your prognosis now? You've seen your audiograms, what kind of hearing do you have left.

Vinell Lacy: I just had the test a week ago and found that one ear is almost completely no hearing left. The other one's about 30%. I have been recommended by two doctors to get a cochlear implant.

Richard: That's interesting. Now my question is, we've had conversations before about this, but it was a long time ago. And your feelings about cochlear implants back then where you're ready, and you may not be ready today, but I'd like you to talk about what you think the pros and the cons are of getting a cochlear implant at this point.

Vinell Lacy: Well, that the cochlear implant is a great technology. I think that from my experience in the Hearing Loss Association, a lot of my friends and the board members have the cochlear implant. I am just at this point undecided. I'm not ready to go there yet.

Richard: Is there a reason why or bunch of reasons why?

Vinell Lacy: There's a lot of reasons why. If you ask me today, it's because I feel like I do not have the time to take to do it. I did decide to do it in November, I went and had all the tests, got qualified, set up the surgery, and had a small car accident that affected the right side of my head, and the doctor wouldn't do the surgery at that point. I was like, "Is this just telling me not to do it yet." I held it off, and now I'm just not ready.

Richard: Okay, that makes sense. You have a young child and have medical emergencies. How do you feel about not being able to grab a phone and make a call or talk to the doctors yourself? How do you deal with that?

Vinell Lacy: It is devastating. It is devastating. My only son was in ICU for three months and you could not get any information unless you called, and I was unable to do that.

Richard: What did you do?

Vinell Lacy: I had to depend on someone else to make the call, to talk to them, and that doesn't seem personable. It's heartbreaking to be able to get secondhand information about your son or anyone in an emergency. We are not even able to call 9-1-1 and be able to hear on a phone, and when they start asking you questions and you can't answer them, it's really devastating.

Richard: How would you handle it if you need to make a 9-1-1 call. Let's say you're home alone, somebody trying to break-in, what do you do to communicate mostly?

Vinell Lacy: Mostly e-mail or text.

Richard: You can't take a phone call.

Vinell Lacy: At one point I had to make a 9-1-1 call.

Richard: What happens there.

Vinell Lacy: And I called 9-1-1 and they kept asking me questions and I kept telling them the situation, and they kept asking me questions.

Richard: Did you tell them you were deaf, and you couldn't hear them?

Vinell Lacy: I told them yes. I said, "Listen, I'm hard-of-hearing, I am not understanding your questions, this is where I live, and I need a policeman now," and she just kept asking me questions. And I screamed louder, "I cannot understand what you're saying, I need someone here now!" And finally, she just kept talking to me.

Richard: And what happened in the end? Did they send anybody?

Vinell Lacy: They just showed up and in person I could talk to them.

Richard: In other words, you wasted time because- Vinell Lacy: I could not hear.

Richard: I need to go back a few steps. You were in your 30s when you finally got a hearing aid and realized you had the hearing loss. Do you have any siblings or anybody in your family with hearing loss too?

Vinell Lacy: My mother has hearing loss and there are six children, and three out of six have the same hearing loss that I-

Richard: So, genetic component to it. What kind of hearing aid are you using now?

Vinell Lacy: I'm using a Phonak.

Richard: Do you get good results with it?

Vinell Lacy: I am a lot better with the hearing aid than I am not. And without my Icom that I normally use, I cannot answer the phone at all. I cannot hear anything. With the Com Pilot, I'm able to make a familiar voice. I think when you get a severe hearing loss like we have, we learn to hear some things and some voices.

Richard: When you're 30 you lose your hearing. Were you isolated from your family or your friends? I know you told me about your business side, what about your family side? What happened there?

Vinell Lacy: Well, my mom lived out of town and of course I'm the only family member that had moved from home. And yes, I could not talk to them on the phone like I like to, and my mom and dad was getting older. It hurt that you couldn't even talk to them on the phone. So yes, it was devastating. You feel really isolated away from your family. But with my job, we had meetings and met with the judges with the judicial system. I couldn't do it because I couldn't hear in a crowded room. I couldn't hear in meetings. I just did not go to them. I got isolated in my work also.

Richard: What about now, because now you're using hearing aids and you're about to go to a meeting with about 30 or 40 people. How do you deal with hearing in that situation now?

Vinell Lacy: Well once I got with the Hearing Loss Association and I learned a lot of techniques, and I learned to be proactive and tell a lot of people that I have a hearing loss. "Look at me, talk directly to my face," things like that. I learned to fill in a lot. So upset all the time, because before you just feel like no one understands you. And having hearing loss, I feel that a lot of us felt like people thought we were dumb instead of just hearing loss, because the way we look at people and we may answer you wrong. It's really a tough world out there.

Richard: It's a tough world all right. After the American Disabilities Act passed, was anything there helpful to you in your life in terms of business or travel or getting around? Was anything specific under the American Disabilities Acts that you've used or that you're aware of?

Vinell Lacy: I've used a few. The airport has been really devastating. I've missed flights before because they've called my name when they move the gate. But now I go to the desk, and I tell them, "I have a hearing disability. If you do move the gate or any changes to my flight, come directly to me." They have been very helpful in that. The last place I worked; they did supply me with all the special phones. Any hearing device I needed; they supplied it for me. So yes, I've used a few.

Vinell Lacy: They were supportive, but it still didn't get me through.

Richard: Do you listen to music anymore or is music too difficult?

Vinell Lacy: I cannot listen to music and that is very devastating.

Richard: You miss it.

Vinell Lacy: I miss it horribly.

Richard: But you can't hear it. Vinell Lacy: I cannot.

Richard: You're on the fence still about a cochlear implant, I understand that. Is there an event that would make you change your mind and get a cochlear implant tomorrow, or is there something you're waiting for? I'm trying more to find out more about your feelings about them because a lot of people are in your situation, and I want to share how you feel. If you would go ahead and do it tomorrow if something came along you needed.

Vinell Lacy: I don't know how to answer that for sure. If I knew that I could get through the whole process and get to the next level and be able to hear, yes, I would decide for the cochlear implant.

Richard: How would you have doubts though?

Vinell Lacy: My doubts are, and I know this sounds ridiculous, but my life is very busy with family, with sickness. I just feel like I am not mentally ready to go through that process.

Richard: That makes a lot of sense. That makes a lot of sense because no one should be doing this unless they're a 100% into it.

Vinell Lacy: Exactly. Just for instance, I mean I don't want to put my personal life out, but when I scheduled to have the cochlear implant, I was ready. I thought I had the time. I've set everything aside; I'm going to do this because I really feel I need to. That was in November I was supposed to have the cochlear. I lost my mother in November, then of course my son got sick in December and was in the hospital for three months, I lost my dad in March. I feel that I would not have had the time to take for that process and it would have been devastating to me. Now everything's coming around and getting to be calmer in my life, and I am reconsidering the option.

Richard: Because it does take time for rehabilitation. It does take time to commit. There's no question. Then your case fate stepped in.

Vinell Lacy: [crosstalk 00:17:48] Yes. I think you have also must be mentally ready for the cochlear implant. You must set your mind and your time to do what is needed, to get through the process, to make it work properly.

Richard: My last question to you was this. If you had a cochlear implant and your hearing came back to a usable level, is there something you would do differently right now in terms of your business, your family? Have you ever thought about it?

Vinell Lacy: Everything.

Richard: Everything's a big word. Could you [crosstalk 00:18:21] something you'd specifically tell us?

Vinell Lacy: It would. If I could hear today, it would change my world.
Richard: Is there something specific that you could tell?

Vinell Lacy: Specific. I think specifically I would be able to get my business back on track and be able to get back into the workforce.

Richard: That's great. I thank you for your time.

Vinell Lacy: Thank you and you're welcome.

Chapter 20 Mike Dailey

The Unstoppable EMT Mr. D with Bilateral Cochlear Implants

I have seen glimpses of Mike Dailey, the fireman with bilateral cochlear implants. His story seemed to peek out now and then on social media from time to time.

Until he joined the Facebook group, Bilateral CI Warrior, I had been unable to contact him.

Now I have his interview, and this is why is it so important that candidates and recipients take time to listen to it or read the transcript.

Mike embodies the concept that if you have talent, a cochlear implant is not an impediment to accomplishing your dreams. He is a shining example of that.

Many times, I have seen people post the question: What kind of job can I look for if I have a cochlear implant? As Mike tells it, there are no limits. Zero. Nada. None.

Inspirational does not begin to describe Mike Dailey.

Listen or read and learn.

Richard: Good evening. Tonight, we're talking to Mike Dailey, a fireman. I'm going to ask you to state your name, today's date, and where you're at.

Mike Dailey: My name is Mike Dailey. Today is March 17th, 2022. Happy St. Patrick's Day. And I am in Pendleton, Indiana.

Richard: Mike, tell me a little bit about your background, when you lost your hearing, and a little bit more about growing up with a hearing loss and so on and so forth.

Mike Dailey: As a young child, I had chronic ear infections. Today, they would give you tubes. They didn't really do that. I grew up in a rural community. They didn't see any need for it. By the time I was in high school, I had a noticeable hearing deficit, so I started learning how to read lips in trying to overcome that.

Mike Dailey: I aspired of a career in the military, and through an uncle who also had hearing loss that was in the military, back then they used to do a timed test. I knew if I hit the button every six seconds, I would pass the hearing test. So that's how I got into the Marine Corps. While I was in the Marine Corps, I had an incident with a mortar round that landed a little too close, ruptured both of my eardrums, but did substantial damage to my right eardrum and right inner ear. Or middle ear, I guess you would say. After that, I couldn't pass the hearing test.

Mike Dailey: I learned to fake it a little bit more, learned more lip reading, other ways to compensate. Got out of the Marine Corps and got into EMS at the local hospital, became an EMT, and was doing that with aspirations of getting on the local fire department. And was doing well compensating. Became very sensitive to vibrations and feeling. And learning how to, like I said, read body language and things like that, people didn't notice I missed as much. I got hired at the fire department and they sent me down for my physical and I failed. So that was the end of that dream, or so I thought.

Mike Dailey: I went to work for a sheriff's department because they didn't have a hearing test. I was able to fake it for several years and did okay.

Then they opened a prison in the town that I lived in at that point, and they offered me a substantial pay raise to go work at the prison. I did that. At the prison, they figured out I could fix things, so I became the locksmith for the prison. I was on the emergency response team, and they started noticing I was missing radio calls. A lot of radio calls. And they said, "Hey, you need to go get your hearing checked or you're not going to have a job." At the ripe old age of 30, I got my first set of hearing aids. Part of what made that okay was I was a new father, and I couldn't hear my daughter cry. The hearing aids helped.

Mike Dailey:

My hearing progressively started getting worse. I just kept going from one hearing aid dispenser to another. The ENT I was going to said that I had otosclerosis, and he had the same thing, and I had tympanosclerosis. They tried to do a tympanoplasty to fix my eardrum, and it failed because of the hardening of the inner ear. They just kept bumping up the hearing aids and BTEs, behind the ear superpowers.

Mike Dailey:

We moved in that timeframe, and I made friends here in town, and one of them happened to be a professor of audiology at Ball State University. I started going to Ball State and was getting my hearing aids through there. I interacted with her quite a bit. She's like, "You do really well in the booth, but you're not doing so well here in a social setting." She took me back to the booth and turned my chair around and turned the lights out, and I failed miserably. I lost all of my cues. She's like, "Hey, your hearing's a lot worse than what we've thought. It's time for you to see a specialist."

Mike Dailey: I was fortunate enough to... Indiana University Medical here in Indianapolis has a phenomenal ENT, so I went to see him. And he's like, "You have both conductive and sensorineural loss. I think a bone-anchored hearing aid would work for you." We tried the bone-anchored hearing aid, and it was amazing. It crosses over, so I had a hearing aid in one side and a BAHA in the other, and it was really phenomenal. Unfortunately, because of how much sensorineural loss I had, they had it cranked all the way up. It was a BAHA 5 Superpower by Cochlear. And with the button that stuck out, the snap, it vibrated so much that it didn't seal, the skin didn't seal around it.

Mike Dailey: In the meantime, I had gone on from being the locksmith for the prison to being a contractor. Contractor came along, offered me a lot of money. Welder, fabricator. I'm still doing the same thing; I was just making more money and didn't have to deal as much with the inmates. But because of the environment that I worked in, the sweat, the dirt, and everything else, I kept getting infections. The year and a half mark, they pulled that BAHA and put another one in. Went about another year with the second BAHA and started getting the infections again. And he says, "No, this isn't going to work. You're just not getting what I want." Mainly because in that timeframe, my cat quit purring. Evidently, the cat really didn't quit purring, but to me it quit purring because I couldn't hear it anymore. My loss had progressed to that point, and they did the evaluation, and I was a candidate for that ear.

Mike Dailey: They removed my BAHA in February of 2020. I was scheduled for surgery for March 25th, 2020. We all know what happened there. Finally, about July, they opened up the surgery schedule and they got me in, and I got my first implant. A month later when they activated me, it was a whole new world. I guess I had what they called the rock star activation. I was able to understand words instantly. It was phenomenal. I was listening to music on the way home after activation and enjoying it. So that was really neat.

Mike Dailey: I still had the hearing aid on the left side. About six months into it, I was like, "Hey, I'm not hearing as well. I think I need another mapping." Well, they checked the hearing in my left here and they were like, "Hey, your left ear's not working. It's just only good for holding on your sunglasses." They scheduled me for surgery, and I became bilateral. At that point, everybody, my immediate family, my friends, everyone noticed a huge difference.

Mike Dailey: The local volunteer fire department... We call it volunteer. We're practically full-time here because we average about 2,500 runs a year. The local fire chief wanted some specialty training equipment built because they didn't have the budget to buy it. I started working with him and he's like, "Hey, didn't you used to do this?" And I'm like, "Yeah." And he's like, "Well, why don't you do it anymore?" And I'm like, "Well, I've got these." And he's like, "I don't care. I need people." He brought me on to the fire department and I discovered, through research and talking with people, that they had stethoscopes that connected to the phone which connect directly with the cochlear implant. I could hear blood pressures and breath sounds and everything through a stethoscope again. And I got back into EMT class, and I graduate in two weeks.

Richard: We got to have to have a party for you. We're going to have a virtual party. I need to go back a couple steps because your story is just incredible. When you were in the Marines and you had the mortar round explode, did you develop tinnitus from that as well?

Mike Dailey: Horrible. I still have it. It doesn't go away. Without my implants, I think the last time they tested, noise had to be at 180 decibels for me to know it was there. I'm essentially deaf without my implants.

Richard: That was the same thing for me. You could fire a gun behind my head, I wouldn't turn around.

Mike Dailey: Nope. I don't hear anything.

Richard: Now, in addition to your career, the reason I'm going back a little bit is I have mentored veterans, both combat and non-combat, and the issue was if you did not have a hearing loss on your military records, the Veterans Administration would not step in and help. Was that the case when you were there?

Mike Dailey: Yes. When I was in the Marine Corps, I played with a couple different units. Back in 1996, there was a unit called Joint Task Force Six. We did counternarcotics. It skirted the Posse Comitatus. When they shut that down, about a month later, there was a fire at the records repository in St. Louis. I have my DD214. At a certain point, it became useless to fight to me because of the level of care that I could find outside of the VA matched what I wanted to do. To me, it was just easier to get things to make my life better than to fight.

Richard: I want to go back to that one last question because we're going to move forward from here. I've talked to experts from the VA regarding tinnitus, and people who have lost limbs and IEDs and hearing as well. And they say that the tinnitus is worse than the loss of a limb, it is so bad.

Mike Dailey: I could definitely see that. There's never any quiet.

Richard: Now I want to jump forward because you've answered my questions on that. My questions are the chief of the volunteer fire department said to you, "I need a warm body that knows what the hell they're doing." And they were happy to have you. Now, a few weeks ago or months ago, there was another post on the Facebook site with a gentleman who was a fireman, but believed he would get fired if he revealed he had a hearing loss. Now, your experience, you're in a occupation that's dangerous with team members that depend on you. Could you talk a little bit about that? How you deal with that?

Mike Dailey: The NFPA actually has strict rules about full-time firefighters and hearing loss. My chief in particular is working with the state fire marshal to try to get that lessened because they are finding that firefighters are trying to hide their hearing loss, and that's proving to be more dangerous than having people with augmented hearing. They're trying to basically bring them up into the 21st century and change the fire service.

Mike Dailey: Our chief is using me as an example. We've learned how to patch the radio in through my phone so that I can hear the radio calls. My department responds to a lot of accidents on the interstate. If you can imagine the highway noise, all the vehicles, fire trucks running, generators running, and people yelling and everything else. The amount of noise is something that the hearing booths can't duplicate. The guys I work with, I tell them, "Hey, if you need something, a hand signal, get my attention." They know what to do. They'll flash a light at me, they'll wave a hand. A lot of it comes down to I just have to have my head on a swivel a little bit more than normal, and we're able to compensate and make up for it. I'm able to actually hear. I actually have guys say, "What'd they say?"

Richard: I know that feeling. I can go into a dinner with 250 people, but because of the accessory, people are always turning to me and saying, "What did they say? What did they say?" I'm the deaf guy in the room and I'm interpreting for them.

Mike Dailey: I'm always ask them, I'm like, "Do you want me to ask my friend Ray Charles what he saw?" My goodness.

Richard: Now, the other aspect of what you told me before I find fascinating, because I've done the same thing myself, is the bluffing. I believe that most people with a hearing loss, they bluff. Tell me how you worked your way out of that. Tell me how you dealt with it. How did you stop bluffing?

Mike Dailey: It took me a while. The electronic voices were easier to get used to and become more natural than the constant strain of watching people's faces, watching their lips. I think the only reason I was able to break away as much from lip reading was because it was during the pandemic, and everybody wore a mask. I still have to deal with that because we still wear masks in the patient situations and hospitals are still wearing masks. Getting over the bluffing was a lot easier because there's no way to bluff when somebody's wearing a mask. You've got to figure out what they were saying. It was easier transition for me because of that situation.

Richard: I find that interesting because I used to be able to lip read conversations from 25 feet away. After I got cochlear implants, I've lost that skill. I can lip read somebody I'm talking to, but I can't eavesdrop on a conversation anymore.

Mike Dailey: How do I want to say this? My family still tries to get away from me. They figure since I can hear, they can whisper. One, I can catch a lot of the whispers, but two, I keep that lip reading because I try to catch them. Because boy, they set me up.

Richard: How many children do you have?

Mike Dailey: Two daughters.

Richard: Excellent. They have you wrapped around their little finger, I'm sure.

Mike Dailey: Oh, no. No, no, no. Not at all.

Richard: Now, so let me ask another question. Your skills, your abilities, are amazing. What I try to explain to people, or my experience of talking to people, is that if you have a talent, a cochlear implant should not hold you back from going for the job you want. Can you talk about that a little bit?

Mike Dailey: I'm the type of person that if I want to do something, I'll set my mind to do it and I'll just do it. When I did lose the ability to listen through a stethoscope, that was really hard for me, and that was something I missed for several years. Because with the hearing aids, when I first got them, they didn't have the Bluetooth, they didn't have all the technology that we have, so it was a big blow. When I was offered the opportunity and saw the technology, I was blessed to be in a situation where there was somebody that was willing to give me a chance. I wasn't going to let this hinder me. It was going to become my leg up, so to speak.

Mike Dailey: My daughter has a leaky valve in her heart. I can actually hear that with my stethoscope now. There's a lot of other people around that can't with a regular stethoscope. They have to have something to augment it. To me, it's almost a... In the back of an ambulance, people have trouble hearing with a stethoscope with the road noise, the sirens, and everything else. With me, it's a blessing because it tones everything out, and all I can hear is that I can focus on what I'm trying to do. To me, my hearing loss now is not necessarily a hindrance, but it's my leg up in the world. And plus, when I travel on vacation with the family, I can sleep in a hotel a lot easier than they can.

Richard: We had a lightning storm two nights ago here, and my wife said it was the worst storm she's ever heard. I slept right through it. I had no clue.

Mike Dailey: You understand exactly where I'm coming from. It's a superpower.

Richard: We have another podcast interview here on the site with Suzanne Tillotson, who is an intensive care nurse during COVID, and her stories were remarkable. But I remember asking her about listening to her heart. She said she had to listen to special recordings for a long time so that she could differentiate the different heartbeats. There are techniques out there. I think there are quite a number of people in the medical profession, or aspiring to be nurses or doctors, who come to these sites wanting to know their limitations. Your interview here is going to be very, very important for them to understand there are no limits.

Mike Dailey: Definitely not. I try to tell people the only limitations are the ones you set on yourself. This is a blessing. I joke with the guys around here. As they get older, their hearing's going to get worse. As I get older, my hearing's going to get better.

Richard: It's true. It's true. Mike, let me ask you, do you have any last words or words of advice for our listeners before we sign off?

Mike Dailey: The only advice I could give anyone that would really help is don't give up. You can do it. Don't hesitate. The longer you put things off, the more you're going to miss. The amount of things that I have gotten back, hearing the ocean, being able to hear while I'm swimming with my kids, being able to hear my daughter's laughter. That stuff is what's important in life, not what they look like or what can't I do. It's about what can I do. If you look at life of what can you do? How can I make it better? And how can I enjoy this more? Then it's a simple choice.

Richard: Mike, you know what? You're absolutely amazing. I'm so glad you sat down. No, you have no idea, because I've been following your story in and out and different sites, but I've wanted to sit down with you for the longest time. I just want to let you know how much I appreciate your time, how much I appreciate your message. You will be changing lives like you just wouldn't believe from taking time to sit down with me.

Mike Dailey: Well, thank you. I appreciate the opportunity. I've followed you and been a big fan. I think what you do is just awesome. I refer people to your website all the time.

Chapter 21 Rebecca Alexander

Even with Usher Syndrome She Refuses to Fade Away

I was recently given a gift. It was a copy of the book, Fade Not Away: A Memoir of Senses Lost and Found, by Rebecca Alexander, a psychotherapist, who is deaf and blind from Usher syndrome.

It was story I read cover to cover without putting it down. I knew I had to ask her to be interviewed for a podcast.

Many times, the rhetorical question has raised its ugly head: Is it worse to be deaf or blind. Usher syndrome leaves its victim with both.

As Rebecca explains, there is often no timetable for the progression or the degree of the disease. Living under the sword of Damocles, one can be overwhelmed with anxiety or grapple with the problem head on.

Rebecca Alexander is an unstoppable spirit and an extreme athlete. She has summited Mount Kilimanjaro as well as the Inca Trail to Machu Picchu.

As a therapist, her insights to her own condition and those who suffer from chronic complications are invaluable.

Her website is www.rebeccaalexandertherapy.com

Richard: Good afternoon. We are talking with Rebecca Alexander. And just start off by stating your name and where you are.

Rebecca Alexander: So, I am Rebecca Alexander, and I am in Manhattan, New York City.

Richard: I read your book. Actually, your book was given to me as a gift. It was a family that I mentored for cochlear implants, and she gave me your book. And I tore right through it. I thought it was just absolutely fabulous. So, I just wanted to reach out and speak to you.

But among all the interviews I have, you're the first one I have with Usher syndrome. And I know that my listeners would like to know more about your background, about the disease, and then we can go on from there.

Rebecca Alexander: Usher syndrome is the leading genetic cause of deaf blindness in the US and around the world. It is an orphan disease. There are three types of Usher syndrome. A person with Usher syndrome type I is born completely deaf, and they're progressively losing their vision. They usually have balance issues as well.

A person with Usher syndrome type II is usually born with a very sort of specific amount of hearing loss, and they're losing their vision. And they don't generally tend to have balance issues, but they can, and sometimes do, lose more hearing later in life.

And a person with Usher syndrome type III, what I have, experiences the mildest onset of both progressive vision and hearing loss, and have balance issues.

So, when I was diagnosed with Usher syndrome, type III had not yet been identified. So, they told me I had Usher syndrome, but they said they'd never seen it as it presented itself in me. So, it took about 10 years and a lot of researchers, and my family's blood work sent to Helsinki, Finland, where they finally identified Usher syndrome Type III.

It's an orphan disease, and now we have subtypes of an orphan disease, and then we have sub-subtypes, meaning, you can have Usher type 1A, 1B, 1C, 1D, 1F, 2A, 2B, 3A. So, it's definitely an interesting condition to live with.

Richard: You live with a condition, your book Not Fade Away, which is amazing, amazing book, does describe the steps that you went through, and you started to lose your hearing, because obviously, the website is Cochlear Implant Basics, and people who want to know about your hearing. Can you talk a little bit about losing your hearing?

Rebecca Alexander: Yeah. So, interestingly, when I was a child, I used to look at the TV. I used to watch TV by looking out of the corner of my left eye. And I think my family, they just thought it was a funny quirk, that I would my cock head to the side and watch TV.

Well, we learned sometime later, I had what they called a cookie bite of hearing loss. We thought it was because I had frequent ear infections when I was younger. And that was the early onset of Usher syndrome, before we knew that that was what I had.

But my left ear was my stronger ear. So, I had this superimposed way, naturally, of adapting. So, my right ear, I would say, for most of my life, or certainly, when 20s and after, was mostly decorative. It could hear sound, but it couldn't discriminate as well.

But because I had my left ear that was quite strong, I always used my left ear for the phone. If people walked with me, they always walked on my left side.

It wasn't until I was about 19 that I experienced a big dip in my hearing. And I had tinnitus, tinnitus, however you want to pronounce it.

And the sensation was that I couldn't hear people speak to me over it. I suspected that maybe it would go away. And, of course, after about a week or so, it didn't, so I went to a otolaryngologist at the University of Michigan where I attended college, on their medical campus, and that was where they evaluated me.

So, from that time, that really significant dip in my hearing, I was given hearing aids when I was much younger, but I remember the first time I tried hearing aids, and I must have been in, maybe in middle school, and it was just one, for my right ear. And I just remember hearing the fibers of the rug below me and thinking, "This is way too much sound." And, of course, I think there was a lot of feelings of being self-conscious. So, I didn't really start wearing it until I was in college. And then, I was given two hearing aids.

And, so, by the time I was 34, I was tested for cochlear implants for some time, mostly just to get my friends and family off my back, because I didn't really ever think that I was going to be a candidate for a cochlear implant. Remember, there was no trajectory for how my vision and hearing loss was going to progress. So, it's not like I had anybody to look to, to know at what time or my hearing would deteriorate.

But it turns out that, when I was 34, I became a candidate in my right ear for a cochlear implant. I remember collecting all of my hearing aids, and I probably had 15 different types of hearing aids from over the years, that I had used, the blood, sweat, and tears that goes into having amplified hearing. And it was amazing to find that many. I never thought that I'd had that many over that period of time.

So, with a hearing aid, I could discriminate 28% of what was spoken to me in my right ear. And without a hearing aid, I could discriminate 26% of what was spoken to me. So, clearly, that hearing aid was not doing me much good.

256

So, I decided to go ahead and get cochlear implant I'm a psychotherapist by trade. People pay me to listen. But before, I was using a microphone, like an FM system or like a Roger Pen or whatever the mic is that people use. I had one of those that I would sometimes use with my clients.

Richard: Let me ask you a question here, when you're talking about your clients, because, when I lost all my hearing, sudden hearing loss when I was 30, I went into a tailspin. And my psychotherapist, I had to face him, because I had no hearing whatsoever. What kind did you do? Freudian therapy? What kind of therapy did you work with?

Rebecca Alexander: So, I am a psychodynamic psychotherapist. And there's all different types of therapy or different ... There's cognitive behavioral therapy, dialectical behavioral therapy, acceptance and commitment therapy. There's all different types of therapy, Imago therapy, I mean, you name it.

Psychodynamic psychotherapy, in the most simplistic terms, is, essentially, that we are all born and raised in particular families or environments, cultures, socioeconomic status, whatever the things are that we grow up with, those are our primary influences. And we develop at an early age, certain belief systems about ourselves and narratives. And then we grow up, and we're still employing these belief systems or these coping strategies that we developed at a very young age.

The difficulty is, is that because we're still employing these coping strategies or belief systems, as we get older, they're no longer working for us. And not only are they not working for us, but they're also actually working against us and keeping us from being able to make progress and work through some of the real challenges that we have faced. And, so, that is sort of, in a nutshell, what psychodynamic psychotherapy is.

Richard: It's very interesting to me because, following the new Facebook site that we formed back in June, which is Hearing Loss, The Emotional Side, how much people suffer because their families are not supportive of them, maybe not consciously, but they don't know how to face that. They don't know how to tell their families, "Look, just because I have a hearing aid, or a cochlear implant doesn't mean I can hear perfectly again."

And they go into a tailspin. They go downward again. How would you address that?

Rebecca Alexander: Well, here's the biggest difficulty. One of the most important skills we can learn, I believe, is self-advocacy. We often don't learn self-advocacy. I think that, sometimes, when we grow up in families who either are dismissive or aren't necessarily supportive, then it's just a lot of having to try to navigate and figure things out on your own and a lot of feelings of being other, of being different, of being very isolated.

But there's also people who are raised with parents who are very well-intended, but who coddle them, who do things for them, or who don't teach their kids how to self-advocate, which are crucial life skills for anyone, no matter what your circumstances are.

And, so, I do think that there's a spectrum of the type of parenting you see with people who have a hearing loss. But I think that what's most important is, people will say, "Well, why doesn't a deaf person just go and get a cochlear implant? They have a choice to hear. Why wouldn't they choose to hear?"

And that, in fact, is not correct. A deaf person can't just go and get cochlear implant. Hearing is an auditory skill that must be developed at a very young age. It's a muscle. And if you don't develop that skill, then getting cochlear implant may give you some environmental sounds, but certainly not environmental sounds that you can discriminate.

So, when you get cochlear-implanted, there's a whole relearning how-to-hear-digitally process. I personally read books and listened to the audio book at the same time. I actually watched the entire series of Breaking Bad, with the captions on, when I got cochlear implant, to relearn how to hear. So, there's definitely a learning curve.

Richard: I have to remind people all the time that everybody's experience is a little bit different. When you write or when you talk about the fact that maybe you didn't have 100% in the beginning, yes, but 99% of the people getting a cochlear implanted that normalizes with time and with rehabilitation. So, it's something I'd like to remind listeners all the time, not to be discouraged if you hear, "Oh, it doesn't sound normal," because it probably will with time.

Rebecca Alexander: And to your point, Richard, when I first got activated with my first cochlear implant, I thought to myself immediately, "Oh my God, what the heck have I done?" And I say to people, when they're considering it or when they get cochlear implant, if you don't feel that way when you get activated, then something's wrong. It is definitely a process.

And, as you know, I will tell you that sounds sound more natural to me now than they ever have. Our brain is incredibly malleable. And, so, for me, I can recognize your voice from anybody else's voice. But the very first day that I was implanted, I remember hearing the audiologist, and my best friend Alan, who is a man, and the audiologist was a woman, they both spoke, and their voices sounded the same. And it was like, "Hi. How are you? What are you going to do today?"

And I thought I was going to lose my mind. But, of course, even within an hour later, that had continued to evolve. It requires patience. But it is absolutely, in my mind, very well-worth it.

Richard: It's true, because out of the hundreds of people I've mentored or assisted, I can count maybe three or four, who regretted getting a cochlear implant. And those people refused to do any rehabilitation. They thought that it was going to be a magic bullet, and there was no way I could convince them otherwise.

So, yeah, I understand that. But we're-

Rebecca Alexander: Well, that-

Richard: ... talking about whether you go ahead or not, you wrote about your friend, Daniel, who was trying to discourage you from going ahead.

Rebecca Alexander: That was my twin brother. Yep.

Richard: Okay. He was trying to discourage you from moving ahead with it. And you wrote very, very heartfelt paragraph there, about why you moved ahead, why you moved off the fence, and that you still had the fear of the surgery, which, I believe, almost everybody getting a cochlear implant, between the time I was qualified and scheduled my surgery, I made it five months down the road, just to be sure that I was not making a rash decision.

Rebecca Alexander: Right. Everybody has a different process, and I'll tell you, first of all, just to address the people that you worked with who regretted it, I said to myself, "If I'm going to get a magnetic device put into my skull, if I'm going to have something in my skull, then I am going to do everything in my power to get the most out of it."

And I have to tell you, the listening therapy, there are games you can play. I remember my first speech therapist, she had a whole list of those little unknown facts that you find on the inside of a Snapple bottle cap, because they're things that you can't predict necessarily. So, you absolutely have to do the work.

But if you're going to get devices embedded into your skull, then by all means. And I have to tell you, the surgery is not a big deal. I'm not diminishing having to make the decision and go through with it because it's the emotional, I think, aspect of it, that is far more difficult than the actual surgery itself.

Richard: Absolutely. I had two of them done at the same time, so yep.

Rebecca Alexander: Oh, wow.

Richard: That's very rare to do it. But you're true about when you're doing the rehabilitation is so important. I'm a Type A behavior, so I designed my own rehabilitation program. I had no patience for it.

Rebecca Alexander: Of course, you did.

Richard: I understand what you're talking about. I'm glad you had somebody to help you along with it.

One of the things I loved about your book is talking about working your way through the emotional side of moving ahead, which I found very important. So, your book is going to be, obviously, a link will be on this podcast, so I want people to read your book as well.

Can I ask you another question, though, about vision versus hearing?

Rebecca Alexander: Yes.

Richard: Talking about the other side, the vision. How did that affect you?

Rebecca Alexander: I think that, to me, the vision loss has been far more daunting. And this is interesting because, before I was implanted, I used to put my vision and hearing, I would be like comparing having Usher syndrome to a stove, that sometimes my hearing would be on the front burner, and the vision would be on the back burner, and sometimes the vision would be on the front burner, and the hearing would be on the back burner.

If they had what we have for hearing loss, cochlear implants, for my vision, I can't even begin to imagine what that would be like, because it's interesting, the only person I know, and not personally, whoever said that she thought that having hearing loss was worse than having vision loss, was Helen Keller.

And I have always found that hearing loss is very difficult. It's very isolating. There's a lot of shame that comes with it. There are so many ways in which it impacts so many different people, and differently. Some people don't feel that shame. Some people are very stubborn. Some people are very vain, in terms of not wanting to have devices on their ears for people to notice.

But I do think that being able to have that amplification, it's been such a crucial part of this process and has made the hearing loss journey for me all worth it.

Richard: I hope, at some point, that we get some sort of cochlear implant for your vision as well, because-

Rebecca Alexander: Yep.

Richard: ... I know that it would be a tremendous boon. I got to tell you, frankly, I can't imagine, if I had to make the choice, which one I would do. It's incredible.

I'm going to give you the floor, and I'm going to let you tell our listeners anything you want about your journey, about what they should be doing, what you did, because I have to tell you, quite frankly, after reading your book, I find you to be unbelievably remarkable person, and I'm going to give you the floor to talk to our listeners.

Rebecca Alexander: Yeah. Well, first of all, I appreciate that. The book, it's funny because I'm almost 44 now, and so it almost feels ... I'm implanted on both sides. I was only implanted on one side at the time. I got my second implant, I think I must have been 37, my left ear became a candidate.

When I got my first cochlear implant, I remember, I sat in the bathtub the night before, and I cried, and I was massaging my right ear and sort of apologizing to it, in some ways. It's so interesting how we go through the emotions of this process, thanking it for how hard it worked. And it makes no sense really, but it's just a testament to the human condition and the emotions that we experience.

COVID really brought mental health to light. I think it gave it more of a platform than it ever had before, and I'm very glad that it did. But living with hearing loss or vision loss, or whatever the adversity is that you face, to me, is far more difficult from an emotional and psychological standpoint, than it is even from the physical standpoint.

Because I had orientation and mobility training that I learned and how to use a cane, but actually having to go out into the world, to have a coming out, so to speak, as someone who is not disabled, to someone who is disabled, out in the world, that was a real process for me.

Now, that had nothing to do with whether I had learned the physical skills to be able to use my cane in public. I learned all that. It was the emotional and the psychological implications of it, that I had to reckon with and come to terms with.

And the first five, six or seven times I used my cane in public, I cried. And that was what I had to go through, in order to develop the ability to tolerate this new identity, in some way, that I would take on whatever the preconceived ideas are from anybody else who saw me on the street, about a person with a disability.

263

So, to me, people say, "Oh, just get over it," or "Distract yourself," or whatever the things are that people suggest that you do. I mean, people use substances. They drink. They use drugs. They gamble. Sex. You name it. People have all these different vices to not have to feel their feelings or to avoid feeling their feelings.

And, at the end of the day, there is no way to get over anything. You can't move on from anything. You have to get through it, and you have to go through it.

And it's interesting, too, because I say that Usher syndrome is the worst thing that's ever happened to me, and it is the absolute best thing that has ever happened to me. And that coexistence of feeling those two vehemently opposed feelings, beliefs, is a very humbling way to live.

It creates a real sense of just feeling a tremendous sense of compassion for others, a tremendous sense of compassion, even for myself, and an ability to understand that we all are going through something. And no matter how scary something may be, that you can do something that's very scary and overwhelming to you, and also be incredibly afraid.

Richard: Just amazing. It's true. It's true. Because I think you said it best, and you said what you do, as a therapist or helping others, is an act of justice. It's an act of justice, of overcoming the unfairness of the world, I suppose, by helping others. So, it's just an amazing outlook.

I'm going to close this off by asking, I know that people are always on social media, looking for therapists who understand the hearing loss. Basically, when I found a therapist, he had survived leukemia, against all odds, so he understood something from the point, viewpoint that I was dealing with. But finding a therapist who understands hearing loss is almost impossible. Do you do therapy by remote?

Rebecca Alexander: Yes.

Richard: I'll make sure everybody has your contact. You're going to be overwhelmed next week.

Rebecca Alexander: Well, and I think that is, it's just like anything. I sometimes encourage people, if they're having trouble in their area, finding a therapist, let's say someone they want to see in person or someone who is in network with their insurance, I say that if you can't find someone who specializes in hearing loss, try looking for someone who specializes in grief and loss.

Richard: That's exactly the grounds that we formed the Facebook site of The Emotional Side. The question came up, whether hearing loss was a amputation, or if you were grieving for that hearing loss. So, the two people I put it together with, that was the substance of our discussion about grieving. So, absolutely on target.

Rebecca Alexander: It's important, when you find someone, that you may have to educate them a little bit. And that's frustrating because we don't want to have to do that. So, it definitely helps to have a therapist who specializes or who they, themselves, has a hearing loss, so that they really understand it.

But I think that, oftentimes, people are afraid to ask for help because we don't want to feel like we can't do something completely independently. We're taught to be autonomous and independent and not need to ask for help. And part of, I think, what can be helpful, in coming to terms with needing to ask for help is, first of all, we expect people to be mind-readers. We are passive-aggressive, or we get frustrated or angry with a family member or our loved one or friends because they don't do certain things. They don't make the accommodations we want them to. We expect them to know what we need.

And being able to tell people what you need is how you get your needs met. And unfortunately, people are not mind-readers. But another way that

I think you can engender that ability in yourself to ask for help is that, when you ask someone for help, what you're doing is you're telling them, in no unspoken terms, that they matter, and that they're needed. And there is nothing that we want to know more in this life than that we matter and that we're needed. Asking for help is not asking someone to do something for you. I think that's a really important piece for people to remember as well.

Richard: Absolutely. I agree with you 1000%, and you've covered so much. And I'm absolutely thrilled you took the time to talk with us. So, let's say goodbye. Wish you a happy holiday.

Rebecca Alexander:

Thank you.

Richard:

And you'll hear from us again, I'm sure.

Rebecca Alexander:

Oh, I so appreciate it. Thanks for taking the time with me today.

Chapter 22 Isabella Rodriguez

Her Transition from a Cochlear BAHA to the Osia

Many who begin their investigation about cochlear implants are confused about the differences between cochlear implants and a device called a BAHA (Bone Anchored Hearing Assistance or Aid). They are under the impression that they can choose between these interchangeably.

The BAHA and the cochlear implant are designed for very different types of hearing loss and only the ENT or surgeon can make the determination based on a battery of tests.

I was fortunate to be introduced to Isabella Rodriguez, a recipient of a BAHA since the she was three months old. Her journey has been remarkable. She is amazing and explains the stages of her hearing loss and her decisions to make the best of her life. In fact, she is an inspiration and a prime example of an unstoppable dynamo.

I see nothing but a brilliant future for a very articulate and caring person. I am glad she took the time to talk with me.

Richard: Good morning. This morning we're talking to Isabella Rodriguez, who is a user of a BAHA, B-A-H-A, better known as a Bone Anchor Hearing Assistance or Bone Anchor Hearing Aid. It's used for a different type of deafness, and I know when people come to our site, I've

267

often seen confusion between using a BAHA and a cochlear implant. So, I'm going to let Isabella tell her story first about her journey, how she lost her hearing, and we'll move on from there.

Isabella Rodriguez: Good morning, Mr. Richard. Thank you so much for having me today. I'm Isabella Rodriguez. I'm 21 years old and I'm currently a senior at the University of Georgia. So, basically, my story starts the day I was born. I was born with conductive hearing loss, and I was born with microtia on my left side, which means absence of an ear. So, basically, when I was born, I was born without an ear on my left side, and I was born with bilateral atresia, which means absence of the ear canal. So, I was born without an ear canal on both sides, which is what resulted in the conductive hearing loss.

Starting at around three months, I started on a Baha Soft Band, and I wore that all the way up through high school until I got to college, and in May of 2021 I received the OCS surgery. It was a very easy, simple, and painless process, and I can now say that I love my OCS device. I wear it every single day. I wear it everywhere I go, and it benefits me in every single aspect of my life.

Richard: Do you wear it on both sides? Two units or just one?

Isabella Rodriguez: I just have it on one side, the left side that had the microtia, but I do plan on, eventually getting the second device on my right side.

Richard: So, you went from the soft band for almost 20 years, and obviously it helped because your speech is excellent. Why did you wait so long to get a BAHA?

Isabella Rodriguez: One of the biggest things was some other medical conditions. Once I was pretty much old enough to say that I did want to transition to surgery, because, like you said, I was doing so well just with the soft band at the time, it was just best for my parents to decide to just let

268

me continue and we'll see once I get older. And just some other health conditions popped up. I had arthritis, so I was on some medications that would've conflicted with surgery. So, once I was older, it was the best decision.

Richard: Now, the Osia is a relatively new unit. Can you describe a little bit about the surgery? Why is it different from the traditional BAHA, which is a post? Tell us a little bit about that.

Isabella Rodriguez

So, the Osia-2 is under Cochlear Americas, and the surgery was very simple, painless, quick. A little joke I like to say is that I was in and out of surgery and back home before some of my friends were even awake to start their day. It was over the summer, so I can give them some credit for that, they slept in, but I went in in the morning, talked to my ENT, my surgeon, and the next thing you know I was awake.

So the Osia, there's an internal device and then an external device, and that internal device is placed underneath the skin and the muscle layers of your head, and they just place it right under and then they close you up. I can't even see my scar. My surgeon did such a good job. She even braided my hair in surgery, so she didn't have to shave any off at all, so I woke up with all my hair. It was amazing. As a girl in college, your hair was very important to you. I had a bandage on my left side for about 24 hours, but then in another three weeks I was activated.

I guess the biggest difference from the BAHA with the post, like you said, is that there's nothing protruding from my skin, and I really like the idea of something being underneath the skin rather than protruding. There's a little bit less of a risk for infection around the area and just the delicacy around the skin that you would get from that post, you don't really get from the Osia.

Richard: Now, I've known other people who have gotten the BAHA and the post is a major issue with them, whether it's infections or bleeding on the pillow, and when they switched to an Osia, those problems disappeared. So, I'm sure... You never faced the post, though. I have a question about music. How do you deal with music? Does it sound natural?

Isabella Rodriguez: Yeah, I love music. I listen to music all the time when I walk around campus when I'm working out. Music has always been there for me. I understand some people who lose their hearing later on in life, they lose their touch with music, but for me, I've been blessed enough to always been able to enjoy it. With the Osia, I can Bluetooth directly from my phone to my Osia, so another joke I like to make is that I never have to buy any Air Pods or headphones, because now it streams directly into the Osia.

Richard: You saved a little money there.

Isabella Rodriguez: Yeah.

Richard: I'm going to be very, very curious if you go for a bilateral setup, because as I understand the BAHA or the Osia is working on vibrations, and I don't understand quite how the left and the right are going to separate those vibrations, because they're going to cross, unlike a cochlear implant where you're going to two sides of the brain directly, there's no real interference. So, I'll be very curious. Now that brings me up to another point. Have you tried using the soft band on the other side?

Isabella Rodriguez: I have not, no. I've grown up with using a device, some sort of hearing technology, on just the one side, so I have never personally been curious. Like I said, I do see myself in the future getting that second abutment, and I'm sure that that's something that my audiologist will help me with, in terms of the crossover. I know that there are a lot of different programming that really try to combat that issue.

Richard: I also am curious because you are among the younger people I've interviewed for my podcast. Can you tell me about growing up with the hearing loss and what school was like, what your friends were like? Was there bullying? Was there support? Tell me a little bit about your early life.

Isabella Rodriguez: So, from as far back as I can remember, preschool, elementary school, even the first part of middle school, for me having the hearing loss was a cool thing. At show and tell I would always just pull off my hearing device to show the entire class. I loved answering questions. I wanted people to ask me questions. No one really cared. When you're a kid, you just want someone to play with. You're not really thinking about those other little things. Were they always in the back of my head? Yes. But were they in the back of other kids' heads? No.

But once I started to get a little bit older, the girls started getting meaner. The bullying definitely did come up in high school. I was on the volleyball team for all four years. It was honestly a horrible experience. They were so mean, tried to use my hearing loss as the reason for our losses, as well as the coach. He would pull me out of the game and say, "Oh, I'm pulling you out because you can't hear me when you're on the court." That was hard.

But as far as support, I have to give all the credit to my mom and my dad. They supported me and advocated for me so much throughout my school years, and I had support from a lot of my teachers that I'm truly blessed for, and that's what I believe made me so successful going through school.

Richard: So, you were in high school and that's really when the troubles started?

Isabella Rodriguez: Yes.

Richard: The hormones kick in and everybody gets mean. I get it.

Isabella Rodriguez: I guess so.

Richard: My question now is about you're in college now. Tell me about how you chose where you went to school and how do you cope in the classroom? Are the professors supportive?

Isabella Rodriguez: Yeah. Yeah. Actually, my college experience is a little bit unique and not only because I've been a college student through Covid 19, that was unique in itself, but my freshman and sophomore year I was a student at Gallaudet University in Washington DC, and I was on the volleyball team there, as well. Gallaudet University is a deaf university in Washington DC that caters to the deaf and hard of hearing community. All of my classes were instructed in American sign language. So, I actually went there a month early to have an immersive program in learning the language and learning the deaf culture. And honestly, that is where I gained 90% of my confidence in regard to my hearing loss, because, as I said, in high school I went from not really noticing a difference between other students to all those mean kids. The bullying really tore my confidence down, but I gained it all back in Gallaudet. And there having hearing loss, it doesn't matter because everything is in American sign language.

I truly loved the school, but with Covid 19, I ended up transferring to the University of Georgia, and that's when I really started to have to advocate for myself again. So, I reached out to the Disability Resource Center, set up interviews and meetings with my advisors there. They asked if I needed note taking if I needed pre-recorded lectures. At the time during Covid, I did take all of that. I also asked for preferential seating in the classroom. But with the University of Georgia being as big as it is, you just walk into the classroom, and you get to sit wherever you want. So, I would always choose to sit up at the front.

And with the Osia system I get this thing called a Mini-Mic. It's part of my Disability Resource Center accommodations. But the teachers, the professors, have to wear them if I give it to them. So, at the start of every class, I come in about three to five minutes early, and I place it on their desk, and they know that if they want to walk around the class they need to wear it, or if they're going to just stay at one spot to teach the class that they can just leave it on the podium or on their desk.

Richard: Now that's interesting, because I have spoken to or mentored college students before, and when a professor is uncooperative, and it happens from time to time, their resentful of having to make accommodations, did you experience that at all?

Isabella Rodriguez: Personally? No. I think we've come a long way just as a society to be more accepting of people with certain conditions maybe need a little more extra help here and there. So, I've been very lucky. Again, I've been taught from a young age to advocate for myself and to be very straightforward with what I need to be successful. Because for me, I don't play around with my education. I want everything to be accommodated to me because I need them. So, I do try to advocate the best I can for myself.

Richard: Do you use anything like speech-to-text apps when you're in the classroom? Do they work for you?

Isabella Rodriguez: I personally don't use those, no. The Mini-Mic is really helpful for me, because it's that direct streaming into the Osia, so I can hear the teacher's voice as if I could hear them through Air Pods or anything like that.

Richard: So, you're very lucky you live in an age where they're accommodating disabilities. When I went to school, I graduated almost 50 years ago, trust me, there was nothing like that. My next question, it has to do with the decibel differences. Do you think there are going to be differences on each side of your head if you got a second one? Have they talk to you about that?

Isabella Rodriguez: Yeah, so there is more of a higher degree of loss in the left ear, which is the ear that is already implanted, rather than the right side. So, there is a difference of decibels between the two ears they have talked about. I would actually get a better gain, even though I can hear a little bit better out of the right side, if I were to get that second device. As I said before, that is 100% something that I would talk to my audiologist about in as far as the programming and setting everything up goes.

Richard: This has been very, very interesting, and I'm sure it's going to be very helpful to people who want to know the difference between the BAHA and the cochlear. The fact that you're basically missing the outer and the middle ear is a problem, which is why the BAHA is required in your case. If people want to reach out to you who are candidates, do you have any problem with that?

Isabella Rodriguez: I would love that.

Richard: Good. You're like me. We help. We feel better by helping people move forward.

Isabella Rodriguez: Yes.

Richard: What are you studying, by the way?

Isabella Rodriguez: I'm studying audiology.

Richard: Good. Great.

Isabella Rodriguez: Surprising enough. I just finished my fall semester of my senior year in undergrad, so I'm in the process of applying to my graduate programs.

Richard: Are you going to be doing graduate programs in Georgia or are you looking at other places?

Isabella Rodriguez: So, that's the crazy thing. There are no audiology graduate programs in the State of Georgia. I'm very lucky to be attending

274

the University of Georgia, but I'm not very lucky of being an in-state student in Georgia, because I'll have to pay out of state tuition next year for wherever I decide to go.

Richard: I think you'll come on down to Florida. I think we have plenty of graduate studies in audiology down here.

Isabella Rodriguez: Yeah.

Richard: The University of Miami would be fabulous for you.

Richard: All right, before we close the interview, is there anything you would like to tell the audience about your background, about the future, about anything at all? The floor is all yours.

Isabella Rodriguez: I guess my biggest lesson out of all of this is that you get to choose your own identity and you get to choose how you carry yourself in life, and although hearing loss is something that sets you apart, it sets you apart in the unique way. You get this whole new perspective on life that everyone else will never understand. It's such a small community, and it's important to find comfort and confidence in the small community that you now belong in. And to always hold your head up high and just remember that there's nothing that you can't do that someone with typical hearing can. There's so much technology, there's so much support, there's so much information out there to help everyone involved.

Richard: Isabella, I have to tell you, you are amazing.

Isabella Rodriguez: Thank you.

Richard: I really appreciate your time. If you move forward with the second side, we'd love to keep track of how you're doing, whether you do it or not. Thank you so much for your time today.

Isabella Rodriguez: Thank you.

CHAPTER 23 OLIVIA ROSE ALLEN

THE SKY IS THE LIMIT. LITERALLY.

As soon as I finished recording this interview with Olivia Allen, I started searching for local flying instruction. Why? Because she reminded me of a long forgotten item on my to-do list from my pre-cochlear implant days; to learn to fly.

At the time, deafness intimidated me from accomplishing anything that required hearing. After listening to this remarkable cochlear implant recipient, I was inspired to accomplish that goal.

Deaf from birth, Olivia received a cochlear implant at eleven months of age.

Since that time, as she noted in the interview, "The sky is the limit."

Working her way to obtain a commercial pilot's license, I think her story will inspire others to reach for their goals. A cochlear implant is the tool you might need to achieve your dreams.

Richard: Okay. We're talking to Olivia Allen today. Would you please state your name, the date, and what city you're in?

Olivia Rose Allen: My name's Olivia Allen, today is April 1st, 2022, and I am in Indiana.

Richard: Tell me a little bit about your hearing loss? I'm going to have a lot of questions after you give your introduction.

Olivia Rose Allen: I was born deaf. It took my parents realizing that I failed my hearing test to realize that I was deaf. And it was still a couple weeks after that before they actually realized I was deaf because the nurses told them that I had failed the test. But that it was likely just clogged with the stuff that you have after you're born. They realized that nothing was soothing me because I couldn't hear anything, so that's when I became deaf.

Richard: How old were you when they realized you had a problem?

Olivia Rose Allen: Oh, I was born deaf, so they knew right away.

Richard: Were they in denial or did they get help for you right away?

Olivia Rose Allen: Oh, they helped me right away, but I didn't get my surgery for cochlear implants until I was 11 months old.

Richard: Why'd they wait so long for that?

Olivia Rose Allen: I got my surgery done in 2001 and they didn't do surgeries that young, so I was the youngest at that time. Then like a month later they did six month old.

Richard: You had them done one at a time or two at the same time?

Olivia Rose Allen: I just have one cochlear implant on my right.

Richard: And you never considered one for your left side?

Olivia Rose Allen I don't have a cochlear implant for my left side, no.

Richard: Do you have a hearing aid in the left side or no hearing there?

Olivia Rose Allen: Just the cochlear implant on the right side and nothing else on the left side.

Richard: Okay, I think people will be curious why not? Is there a medical reason or you just prefer not to have that?

Olivia Rose Allen: It's been so long that I just never really wanted another one, and I was doing perfectly fine with one. I just decided to stay with one cochlear implant.

Richard: Tell me a little bit about your time in school? Were you able to function well? Did you go to mainstream school or special school?

Olivia Rose Allen: At age three, I went to St. Joseph Institute for the Deaf in Indianapolis. Before they opened in 2001, the Director, Teri Ouellette, she was working with me before then. I was actually the first student enrolled in that school even though I wasn't going to St. Joseph's at the time. But after I went there, I had mainstreamed to public school in kindergarten and then stayed there until I became a senior, so 12th grade. And it was a small school, so it was just one school the entire time.

Richard: Then you developed a passion for flying. How did that come about?

Olivia Rose Allen: My uncle was an air traffic controller in South Bend, Indiana and Elkhart, Indiana, and they had a day where you could go out as a child to go fly with a pilot for like 15 minutes. It was called Young Eagles. The pilot asked me if I wanted to sit in the front seat with him and I said, "Yeah." I went up with him and decided that I loved it. I was probably like 10 or 11, maybe 12 years old at the time. I'd always been obsessed with airplanes. Like I would watch them in the sky all the time, and if my dad saw an airplane or my mom saw an airplane, they always pointed it out because they knew I was obsessed with them.

Olivia Rose Allen: But it wasn't until my 10th grade year that I really decided, "Oh, that's what I want to do." So right now, I'm in school for that and I'll have my private license in less than two months and then my commercial license in about a year after that. At some point, I'll have to get my flight instructing license to teach other people how to fly so I can get my hours in for the airlines.

Richard: I've got several questions about the flying. Obviously, the use of the radio, has that become a problem or did you have to learn special techniques to do it?

Olivia Rose Allen: Talking to air traffic control is definitely difficult. They have their own lingo, they talk very fast, and so what I typically have to do is just tell them that I'm a student pilot and they need to slow down. Usually, that works but I have my cochlear set all the way to high, and then I have the Bose aviation headset and that drowns out as much noise as you can get. It's the best headset on the market right now. It definitely helps drown out, but there's definitely times where I don't catch everything, so I have to ask them to repeat themselves.

Richard: Well, there's a question I have for you about you're not streaming, you're listening through the headset like I am now, just with the headset over your processor?

Olivia Rose Allen: Yeah, I took the headset over my processor and hear as best as I can like that. I don't stream or anything like that.

Richard: Okay, because I've spoken to other pilots, now obviously, not as young as you, and they've said that the FAA is allowing more prosthetic devices in the cockpit such as streaming to your headset and all. But that doesn't seem to be your issue at all.

Olivia Rose Allen: No, I actually didn't know that was a thing until recently. I talked to Jordan Livingston, he's also another pilot that has a cochlear implant. As far as I know, he's the only other pilot to get the commercial license with the cochlear implant. But he streams from his cochlear implant into his headset. I didn't know that was a thing, but with the new processor I'll be getting, we're trying to figure out how that's going to work out. If we'll even be able to do that or he'll end up having to do the same thing I do.

Richard: Which processor do you have now? What are you using?

Olivia Rose Allen: I have the Nucleus 6, but I'll be getting the Nucleus 7. As soon as I get my private pilot license, I'm going to get that. So that way it doesn't mess with the process of getting my license just because I don't want to have to spend forever getting used to it. Because it took me like five months to get used to my Nucleus 6 after having the Freedom still.

Richard: Okay, so you have upgraded from one to another because I've interviewed other people who've had their processor, their internal processor for 35 years and now they're on the seventh or eighth generation of external processors. You've been one upgrade since Freedom and now you ready for the N7?

Olivia Rose Allen: Yeah, I'm not sure what the one I had before the Freedom was called, but it was a box that was on my back and that's the one I had for a while. I've been through the system.

Richard: That's fine. I mean, a lot of people are going to be very impressed with the fact you're using the cochlear implant, that you're so young, and you're going to be getting a commercial license. What happens when you get the commercial license? Do you have to go through a period of apprenticeship, or will the airlines hire you?

Olivia Rose Allen: Well, basically, once I get my commercial license, I can be hired. As a private pilot, I can't so this will just allow me to go... If like a skydive company wanted to hire me, they could, or anybody else that they wanted to take a small trip, they could pay for everything, and I would just transport them from one place to another. But, basically, I have to have 1500 hours to go to the airlines. Once I get my commercial, I can build up my hours so that I can get those 1500 hours to go to the airlines.

Richard: How long do you think that might take you?

Olivia Rose Allen: If I become a flight instructor, hopefully, it won't take me more than two or three years to get all those hours. Hopefully, I'll be in the airlines by the time I'm like 26.

Richard: You're absolutely amazing. Did your parents encourage you to go for this or something you just did on your own?

Olivia Rose Allen: You mean as far as the flying part?

Richard: Yes.

Olivia Rose Allen: Well, my parents always told me that I could do whatever I wanted to, so they were very supportive when I told them that I was going to be a pilot. I think it's something they didn't expect, but they also did because they knew how obsessed I was with airplanes. As you can see, I actually have a big old canvas board behind me with an airplane on it. I've just always been told that nothing can stop me unless I let it, so I just go for what I want.

Richard: It's interesting because on the website, one of the things I like to do is find people like you who can encourage others and say to them, "If you move forward and get a cochlear implant, your world opens up."

Olivia Rose Allen: The sky's the limit. But even the moon has footprints on it, so I guess we can't really say the sky's the limit, can we?

Richard: Have you met people who have a hearing loss to severe hearing loss? And did you help them move along to show them what a cochlear implant can do?

Olivia Rose Allen: There's actually a girl in my town in Colfax that has a bilateral cochlear implant. Her parents adopted her from China, so they didn't know anything about cochlear implants. But since I was raised around them, they knew like what their options were, and they actually got her cochlear implant. Then a couple years later she got another one, so she's

281

doing pretty well because they knew about cochlear implants because they had somebody to actually relate to.

Richard: That's important, very important. I think you've told me before; you mentioned you will be doing work with skydivers next summer, I believe, is that correct?

Olivia Rose Allen: Yes, I will be working at the Frankfurt Airport. It's like 10 miles from me and they have a skydive operations, and I'll be bringing people back from the middle of the field, back to the ramp. I'll be doing some office work, and likely, I will be sitting in the co-pilot seat as much as I can to just get some time in an airplane.

Richard: Have you done skydiving yourself?

Olivia Rose Allen: I have, yes. It was pretty fun.

Richard: Did you wear your implant when you went diving?

Olivia Rose Allen: I wore up in the plane, but I handed it to the person that I was strapped to and he put it in his pocket. And then once we reached the ground, that's when I put it back on.

Richard: I was wondering because once in a while people ask the question, can you wear your cochlear implant when you're skydiving? I had no way to know to answer that.

Olivia Rose Allen: If you wore a helmet, you could. But usually the people that are skydiving, the instructor will wear the helmet and you won't. Unless you have your own helmet, definitely do not attempt it.

Richard: That's right. Let me ask you another question, anything you would like to advise young people who are afraid to get a cochlear implant because it'll stick out on their head or will make them look different. Sometimes they're reluctant to move forward because of that. And I would love to know your impressions, what you would tell them about getting the cochlear implant?

Olivia Rose Allen: I can't say whether or not I would've gotten a cochlear implant if I was my age now, and all I knew was sign language. But I'm definitely glad that my parents got it for me because it's opened up so many doors for me. I'm sure people do look at my cochlear and wonder what's going on? But the gift of hearing is so special that I would not be a pilot if I didn't have my cochlear implant. Deaf people, in general, without a cochlear implant, there's only about 300 pilots that are private pilots, but they can only really stick around in the area that they were certified in. Since I have my cochlear, I can go wherever I want and I'm getting my commercial license, so I'll be able to go to the airlines. Anything's possible with the cochlear implant.

Richard: This is very interesting. I didn't realize there were 300 pilots who were deaf. That's brand new to me. They have to stay within sight of the airport or close to.

Olivia Rose Allen: Yeah, so there's an airport near me called Kokomo Airport, and they have a deaf woman who's a pilot, but she's only allowed to stick around locally. She can't go like more than 50 nautical miles. She has to stay in the area just because she can't hear the radio calls and stuff. There are deaf pilots, but there's only one other commercial pilot that I know of that has the cochlear implant.

Richard: Just amazing. You're going to absolutely inspire people to move forward, and I really thank you for your time. Is there anything else you'd like to tell us before we sign off?

Olivia Rose Allen: I would say just don't let anything hold you back. You're in charge of your own destiny, so other people are definitely going to tell you can't do something. My dad's sister-in-law told a bunch of people that I would never be a pilot but here I am, going to school every day so that I can follow my dreams.

Richard: Fantastic. Olivia, thank you so much for your time and the interview, and I'm sure other people have questions and I'll be back to you, at some point, I'm sure. Thank you so much.

Olivia Rose Allen: Thank you. I hope my story will make someone realize that chasing your dreams isn't impossible and they should definitely go for it.

Richard: Thank you so much. Absolutely, I couldn't agree with you more.

Olivia Rose Allen: Thank you.

PART TWO

SURGEONS AND OTHER PROFESSIONALS

CHAPTER 24 DR. JACK WAZEN

A PIONEER AND LEADER IN THE COCHLEAR IMPLANT FIELD TALKS ABOUT YESTERDAY, TODAY AND TOMORROW

I overheard Dr. Jack Wazen mention that the Silverstein Institute, where he is a partner, was in the process of doing the study on vestibular or balance issues in connection with cochlear implant recipients. That topic is of interest to many recipients and candidates of cochlear implants, and I reached out to him to request some time to let him share his experiences and talk more about the study.

His curriculum vitae runs 27 pages of close type. His experience, skills, and his research are simply breathtaking. He's a surgeon trained to restore hearing through a complex and broad range of skills including but not limited to cochlear implants.

I was fortunate that Dr. Wazen agreed to find time in his schedule to sit down for an interview and talk about the study and a wide range of issues relating to cochlear implants; success rates, MRI compatibility, age issues and implant success rates and most of all issues he has faced in his decades of experience as well as his vision and hopes for the future of cochlear implants.

Dr. Jack Wazen: I was on the faculty at Columbia University in New York for many years, was associate professor up there, Director of Otology, Neurotology. I was in charge of the cochlear implant program there. Moved here to Sarasota in 2006. So yeah, I've been here for a while to build a cochlear implant program here. Our program has been growing steadily every year. We have great success with implant program. We're very proud of it.

Richard: Did you originally start doing cochlear implants before you came here or was that something you added on later?

Dr. Jack Wazen: No, I was doing them in New York before I came here.

Dr. Jack Wazen: But Dr. Silverstein, here, was doing cochlear implants before I came.

Dr. Jack Wazen: There were implants performed here before I moved to Sarasota.

Richard: But then you used your skills to become better.

Dr. Jack Wazen: They recruited me here to raise this division to a higher level and to bring it into the future.

Richard: For the past 13 years you've been growing with cochlear implants. It's my understanding, just in the Tampa Bay area, there's something like 350,000 people with hearing problems is huge population here.

Dr. Jack Wazen: Yeah. The incidence of hearing loss, not just in the Tampa Bay area, but all over the world is massive. And it is disheartening to see how many people with hearing loss are not being helped with either hearing aids or cochlear implants.

Richard: And why is that, in your opinion?

Dr. Jack Wazen: There, there are two main reasons for that. One, is denial and people not wanting to be seen wearing hearing devices and so on. And two, is ignorance. People are afraid of implants. They think a cochlear implant is some major brain surgery. We've been asked this question again and again, is this brain surgery? How dangerous this is? How risky is it? And it is none of that. It's a procedure that is done as an outpatient procedure. You don't even spend a night in the hospital with this.

Richard: I understand that. I spend about 40 hours a week on social media. I work in 24 times zones around the world to help create awareness and to bring people together and to say, "if you have a hearing problem and a cochlear implant has been suggested to you, not to be afraid."

Dr. Jack Wazen: Right. And we need people like you and many others who are successfully wearing implants to spread the message that this is not major surgery and that it makes a difference. Because, living in deafness leads to isolation, leads to depression, aggravates potential cognitive decline and dementia. There's a lot of things that happen if you are isolated without hearing and we have the opportunity today to make deaf people hear and yet when you look at statistics, only about five or 10% of people who need implants are getting them.

Richard: I'm going to step into a dangerous territory right here. The question of deaf community versus the hearing community because you just mentioned the isolation of living in deafness and yet the deaf community is very protective of not getting a cochlear implant. Is that changed at all?

Dr. Jack Wazen: I think that's changed a lot. A few years ago, it used to be a big thing. I don't hear much of it anymore and I think there's an understanding that you can communicate with nonverbal ways, you could sign, and you could communicate, and you could be a happy, successful citizen without hearing if this is what you choose. Now, most people who stick to that are born deaf or people who are children of parents who are deaf. But if you are a hearing couple and you have a deaf child, you're doing the best to get that child to hear. There are people who believe in preserving the quote unquote deaf culture, but that's not for everyone.

Richard: I think that number is shrinking from what I've seen. In your opinion, yes or no?

Dr. Jack Wazen: Yes, it is shrinking. What is also shrinking are the schools for the deaf.

Richard: Yes, I've read that, and I understand at Gallaudet University more and more classes have people with cochlear implants there as well.

Dr. Jack Wazen: Yes, and it's all because technology is evolving, and cochlear implants today are not what they used to be. The outcomes and the results and the change of life that they provide is very different.

Richard: What kind of success rate do you see when somebody is implanted? I know there are no guarantees in life, but in your experience, what kind of success would you say on a number basis?

Dr. Jack Wazen: I could predict normally that if I put a cochlear implant in a person, their hearing level, their hearing thresholds are going to be far superior to their preoperative implant levels and they're going to be better than their best hearing aid that they've ever used. That is predictable. What is not predictable? In cochlear implant is the speech recognition. How well can you understand speech with or without visual cues? That's the part that so far, we cannot predict. That depends on how many nerve cells are alive and able to be stimulated by the implant. And we do not have yet a way to measure that before we put in an implant. If you look at the statistics in general, you're going to see people who do extremely well. We've had people, we activate the implant three, four weeks after surgery and on that day they're hearing, and they are smiling from ear to ear.

Dr. Jack Wazen: Like it's a miracle that happened that day. Now, unfortunately not everyone responds like that. And you have people who need to practice listening with the implant.

Richard: Rehabilitation.

Dr. Jack Wazen: Rehabilitation over a period of one or two or three or six months to reach that level of performance. And there's a small group of people who just don't get what we call the open speech, which means understanding me as I'm talking to you. They still need to use visual cues as well as hearing to understand speech.

Richard: Normal people do too.

Dr. Jack Wazen: Normal people do too. Of course.

Richard: One of the other questions people ask me all the time, not only about success, "Will I hear speech again?" But they're also worried about vestibular issues. "Will I get dizziness from this." I see this repeated time after time on social media. I understand you're doing a study or working on a study of vestibular issues and cochlear implants. What can you tell me about that?

Dr. Jack Wazen: The inner ear has two components. It has the hearing part, and it has the balance part and they're interconnected. It's often that you see people who have hearing loss, they also have vestibular problems, balance issues, dizziness issues and so on. Yes, operating on an ear can lead into a temporary dizziness postoperatively. We see that often, but that recovers. And the question that we're trying to ask and answer through our research is how many people who candidate for a cochlear implant have an underlying concomitant balance issue in that ear. Sometimes people have symptoms, some people do not have symptoms yet. And I want to recognize those people before implantation. I want to see how they respond to the implant, and I want to see how does your vestibular system change after implantation?

Dr. Jack Wazen: That's the subject of our study and we're collecting all this data now. We have more than a couple of hundred people that we're studying now. It's a decent number of patients, which allows us to make significant statements. It's not like a couple of patients here and there and then there's no statistical significance to that. No, we're going for good statistical significance.

Richard: How long has that study been going on and when do you expect to have results from that study?

Dr. Jack Wazen: We should have our preliminary data within the next couple of months.

Richard: It's close.

Dr. Jack Wazen: It's close.

Richard: I'm sure everybody listening to this podcast is going to be sitting with bated breath waiting for that one.

Dr. Jack Wazen: I'll let you know as soon as it's out for presentation or publication.

Richard: Another topic that people are very interested in are the MRIs. There are constant battles on social media. "My cochlear implants better your cochlear implant," when it comes to MRIs. But in my experience over the past six months, more and more hospitals are refusing to give an MRI no matter which brand you have. We're here at Sarasota Memorial. Can you tell me a little bit about the protocol? What goes on here if somebody needs an MRI at Sarasota Memorial?

Dr. Jack Wazen: Good question. First, the new implants are all MRI safe. If we implant somebody today they're not going to have any issue in getting an MRI and that's huge. In the past we used to say, "You cannot get an MRI." Just like if you had a pacemaker you could not get an MRI. The fact that you could not get an MRI is not unique to cochlear implants.

However, the industry has changed and now you can get an MRI with a cochlear implant. The question is what the hospital protocol is. Let's not just talk about the hospitals, any radiology place where you go because the hospital does only a small portion of MRIs for the public. There are a dozen other MRI centers where you could go and get an MRI. I've had this discussion with the head of radiology at Sarasota Memorial.

Dr. Jack Wazen: I said, we're getting patients saying, "We're not going to do an MRI because you have a cochlear implant." His response was very understandable. He said, "We have not changed our position that if you have an MRI we're not going to do an implant. However, it's up to you to call us and say, 'this person has an MRI compatible cochlear implant, and we are asking you to do the MRI,'" because they do not want to leave it up to the receptionist who knows nothing about what kind of implant do you have. The safest thing for them to say is "no, with exceptions." So, that's how they do it. Once this generation of old implants is over, that's a different issue. But if somebody calls any radiology office, they will need to research it. How old is your implant? What kind of an implant is it to see whether it's MRI compatible or not? And if it is, is it with the 1.5 Tesla MRI, is it with the 3.0 Tesla MRI? They're going to leave it up to the person and their restorative physician to specifically say what it is, but it's feasible.

Richard: So now they say "no" and you say, "well we can take it out and send you over without the magnet to have an MRI." How often does that happen? Have you done those on? I assume

Dr. Jack Wazen: I have, and I try to avoid that as much as I can because it's not pleasant neither for me nor for the patient.

Richard: Okay.

Dr. Jack Wazen: Yes, you can explant the magnet and put it back in, but you know it's a big deal. You risk infection, wound healing issues and so on. Today all the implants we do are MRI safe, and I hope I'll never have to remove a magnet. If I have a patient with an older implant that needs scanning, I will prefer them to get a CAT Scan with and without contrast it's safe and I don't have to expose the implant to potential trauma.

Richard: I appreciate that. I'd also like to know a little bit more about Meniere's disease because I understand you've had patients with Meniere's disease. Is it preferable to have a BAHA or cochlear implant or depends on the situation? Can you tell me a little bit more about your experience with Meniere's disease and cochlear implants?

Dr. Jack Wazen: Meniere's disease is one of the reasons one loses the hearing to a level that would require a cochlear implant. This difference between being a candidate for a BAHA versus a cochlear implant is a big difference. A BAHA, in this scenario, is to transfer sound from the deaf ear to the better ear. If I put in a BAHA, I'm not reactivating the deaf ear, I'm transferring sound transcranially, through the skull base, so that the good ear is picking up the sound coming into the deaf ear. And that works. It's good. It's covered by Medicare and all insurance. And it's the simplest way to provide a patient with hearing from the deaf side. Cochlear implants' advantage is that they reactivate the hearing in the deaf ear. You are reproducing a two ear hearing situation instead of a one ear hearing. Anytime we can put a cochlear implant in a deaf ear, it is the better option if we have a nerve that is connecting. Somebody who has an acoustic neuroma, for instance, who does not have a nerve is not going to benefit from that. For them, the BAHA is still the answer.

Dr. Jack Wazen: Now, here's the limiting factor is insurance coverage. Because Medicare, for instance right now will not cover a cochlear implant. If you're only deaf on one side, you must be deaf in both ears. If you are dependent on Medicare or insurance, you may be stuck in accepting a BAHA for a single sided deafness situation. If the two ears are out, there's no problem getting a cochlear implant.

Richard: I've understood from my conversations that I've had that Medicare is starting to change that protocol. You haven't heard anything on that scale?

Dr. Jack Wazen: We are requesting and asking and pleading and begging Medicare to change the policies on a bilateral cochlear implant, on single-sided deafness cochlear implants. We have not reached that level of freedom yet. Medicare today will not cover a single-sided deafness person for a cochlear implant

Richard: Not you particularly, is there an organization of doctors that are pressuring Medicare for this? Is there a lobbying group of some sort?

Dr. Jack Wazen: Yes, we are all doing that. The Organization of the Cochlear Implant Association, which basically includes all of us surgeons who do cochlear implants, all the audiologists who program cochlear implants, and the industry of the three main companies. We all belong to that association. They are doing their best to contact Congress, FDA, Medicare, et cetera.

Richard: There was a meeting recently in New Orleans. Was that cochlear implant surgeons or there was convention recently?

Dr. Jack Wazen: Yes. That was the American Academy of

Otolaryngology-head and neck surgery. That's our biggest annual meeting. It's not just for cochlear implants. It's for the whole specialty.

Richard: Okay. My next question for you, particularly, when you decide on a cochlear array, does the candidate choose a company first or do you help the candidate choose which company they're going to go with? What's the surgeon's point of view on that?

Dr. Jack Wazen: We use all three implant companies, and we are happy with all three of them. If you come to me and you say, "I want a Cochlear device or an Advanced Bionic device or a Med-El device," I have

294

no reason to dissuade you or change your mind. In the end you're going to do well with any of these devices. We leave it up to the patient. When the patient is identified as a cochlear implant candidate, we provide them with all the documentation for all three companies, let them study it. Sometimes they come back with questions, sometimes they know what they want. And I've had a couple of patients who would say, "You're the doctor, you decide this is too much for me." And then we could help them with a decision based on need and so on. But you cannot go wrong with any one of them.

Richard: Okay, that's fine. And my question is, do you ever advise candidates not to proceed? Any situations you would say it's not for you?

Dr. Jack Wazen: Yes. I had a patient this morning, she's 68. She was deaf since she was one. She's never used a hearing aid or a cochlear implant all her life. And now 68 years later, they're considering an implant. The potential response and the outcome for somebody who has not been stimulated for so long is not so good. I would say if I put an implant in that person, maybe they will have sound awareness, but they're not going to have any speech awareness. And that person is quote-unquote deaf mute. But she's never heard speech, she cannot speak, will never speak. We have always to put things into perspective in a long period of deafness without brain stimulation is not a good setup for a successful cochlear implant.

Richard: But it can happen sometimes. I had no hearing for 35 years and after I was implanted I got 85% speech. It can happen, but generally...

Dr. Jack Wazen: It can happen. But generally, the odds are not for you. But since you mentioned yourself, did you use hearing aid?

Richard: Yes.

Dr. Jack Wazen: Okay. You are not..

Richard: I didn't use a hearing aid for those 35 years. My hearing went off a cliff when I was 30 so no hearing for 35 years.

Dr. Jack Wazen: And no hearing aid?

Richard: No. I was obviously outside statistical norm.

Dr. Jack Wazen: You're lucky.

Richard: That's why I'm asking you about statistical norms.

Dr. Jack Wazen: Yes. You were on the edge of the statistical norm. You're not in the middle of the bell curve.

Richard: I've been on the edge of everything my whole life. I've asked you about the ones who wouldn't implant. My question is, what's your greatest success story that you can tell me about?

Dr. Jack Wazen: My greatest success story? It's not just one story enough because I've seen it happen more than once is when we turn on the implant and the person is like, "Oh my God, I can hear."

Dr. Jack Wazen: That gives me goosebumps every day. I'll tell you a funny story. We put in an implant on a person, and I see him right after they're activated and then he goes to the bathroom and he walks out of the bathroom and his face is all bright red and I said, "You okay? What's wrong?" He said, "Did you hear that?" I said, "What?" He said, "I went to the bathroom, and it sounds so loud."

Richard: The first time they hear the toilet flush.

Dr. Jack Wazen: The first time he heard himself pee. He walked out embarrassed.

Richard: I have two more questions. One about pediatrics. Do you do pediatric cochlear implants yet?

Dr. Jack Wazen: Yes.

Richard: And they're successful?

Dr. Jack Wazen: Yes, very successful. The age of implantation has been brought down to now one year or even younger. And a child who was born with deafness who is three or five years old, believe it or not, is labeled as too old. Children can be implanted at a young age and when the children are implanted at a young age, they grow up in a normal hearing world. They go to normal schools, and they are main streamed. They are not in deaf schools or in special classes. And that's a remarkable feat.

Richard: And my last question to you is, what would you like to see for the future of cochlear implants?

Dr. Jack Wazen: Education, education, education of the public and of the physicians. There are as many physicians who are ignorant about implants as there are candidates who are ignorant about implants. And I think that's a disadvantage to the public.

Dr. Jack Wazen: I think we try our best to keep educating. We've given talks, we give lectures, articles, things like that. I think better recognition and better acceptance. The ability to put in two implants, I think, would be a good thing. We're born with two ears and for a reason because the brain gets better input from both sides and from both ears. Now, most of the people who get implants get on one side. Fortunately, the other side may have some response to hearing aids. If they don't, then a lot of insurance companies or Medicare would not pay for a second implant on the other side. I would like to see that changed. I would like to see the technology changed so that when we put in an implant, we could always predictably preserve hearing in the implanted ear. Right now, it's not always a predictable thing that we put in an implant that we're going to preserve the natural hearing. We know that the implant will work. The question is can we do an implant and a hearing aid in that same ear?

Richard: The hybrid.

Dr. Jack Wazen: The hybrid style, so that we could stimulate the high frequencies with the implant and the low frequencies with the hearing aid. That's what gives the ear the widest range of stimulation.

Richard: Excellent. I thank you so much for your time.

Dr. Jack Wazen: You're welcome.

Richard: Pleasure. Thank you.

Chapter 25 Dr. Loren Bartels

A Leader in Pediatric Cochlear Implants and Inventor of the Bartels's Kitchen Table Test for CI Qualification.

In 2015 I met with a surgeon and was found qualified for a cochlear implant. I was scared to proceed. I went to seek a second opinion. I sent my records to Dr. Loren Bartels. He took one look at it and suggested, "Why not do both ears?" When I recovered from my shock and thought about it overnight, realized I had nothing to lose, and I agreed. In the end, Dr. Bartels did bilateral surgery on me. I've been grateful and I've tried to play it forward ever since.

I recently learned that Dr. Loren Bartels had performed a cochlear implant surgery on a five-month-old child.

His career with cochlear implants predates the time of FDA approval for them in the United States.

In other words, he has seen and performed surgery and the restoration of hearing through these miracle devices from the start. He talks about his background and the advancement of cochlear implants as well as his own criteria for determining a candidacy. His views on pediatric cochlear implant surgery are invaluable to parents who are seeking answers.

His unique perspective is invaluable to those starting their hearing journey research. I am glad he agreed to take time on his busy schedule to sit down with me for this interview.

Richard: I've been absolutely enchanted with your work, enchanted with what you did for me, but people who are starting out are looking for basic information about what's going on, what to expect from the surgery, so on and so forth. If you could give me a little bit about your background, your education, why you went into the field.

Dr. Loren Bartels: Well, I went into ear work because I was fascinated with ears as a medical student. Back then, we worked on the little hearing bones in the middle ear and that was of like micro-carpentry. So, I've always enjoyed carpentry, and that just was fascinating. But deeper into ear work is very complex physiology, which I also find very fascinating. And then I was fortunate enough in my ear, nose, and throat training to land a fellowship in Los Angeles with the House Ear Institute, and there, Dr. William House was working on cochlear implants on an experimental basis. Richard: How long ago was that?

Dr. Loren Bartels: That was 1979, 1980. So literally, about six to seven years before cochlear implants became FDA-approved, I was helping Bill House doing cochlear implant work in Los Angeles. So again, very fascinating stuff. I did my first cochlear implant in 1986 after the House device became FDA approved. Soon after, the Nucleus first multichannel device became FDA approved and the House device went away, and everyone moved to multichannel. I've been doing multichannel cochlear implants now for 33 years.

Richard: You've obviously seen a lot of changes in the fields.

Dr. Loren Bartels: We have. Initially, they weren't as reliable or anywhere near as reliable as they are now, but reliability now for all of the major manufacturers of cochlear implants now is very high. And what can be done with software with cochlear implants is quite remarkable. There are some ancillary things that are still changing, like Bluetooth connectivity, connectivity to things like Roger systems. There are some things that are happening now that are pretty exciting that help integrate people into groups more effectively.

Richard: Well, the Bluetooth aspect, both for the cochlear implants and hearing aids, is growing drastically. I've seen that happen, and in fact, I had an interview recently with Dr. Victoria Moore and she said the future she saw again was Bluetooth, as great advancements for hearing impaired and for cochlear implants.

Dr. Loren Bartels: Yeah, Bluetooth is making a significant difference. Combining Bluetooth with Roger systems improves ability to understand and moderate noise. If you go to a restaurant that's fairly noisy on a weekend, with a typical cochlear implant or a typical hearing aid, you can get lost pretty easily. But if you have a Roger system, you're more likely to stay connected or at least better connected than you can do without them.

Richard: The same with the Mini Mic from Cochlear, whichever, some of the devices-

Dr. Loren Bartels: The Mini Mic is a lapel microphone and Phonak makes them, ReSound makes them, Oticon makes them, Siemens makes them, a few other companies make them, so depending on the brand of hearing aid you have, you can get a lapel microphone that you can pass around and some of them, it can be a table microphone, and it helps. And it will help up to about 60, 65 decibels. Above that level, it gets overwhelmed, and then the Roger system will work up to about 85 decibels.

Richard: Okay. When you interview a cochlear implant candidate, are they referred to you by an audiologist or how do they come to you?

Dr. Loren Bartels: Most come either from another audiologist or from primary care or from other patients.

Richard: And what's the procedure when you interview a candidate?

Dr. Loren Bartels: Well, first is I can go through what I call the Bartels kitchen table test. The game I play is I have my face turned toward the computer and I speak in a modest voice and see if they can understand me. I don't tell them I'm doing that, but the game I play is, do I perceive them to be severely enough hearing impaired to consider a cochlear implant. And then we go through the usual history and physical exam and review their audiometric studies. If it looks like they might be a cochlear implant candidate, then we put them through a series of testing that we call cochlear implant determination.

Richard: And they go through that test. Now, one of the things those new candidates are overwhelmed with the choice of which company to go with. Do you help them decide or is there a certain criterion that you use to help them or let them decide on their own?

Dr. Loren Bartels: Well, let me first say that we have recently done our own internal study on how well people do with each of the three major companies, and there isn't a significant difference in how well people do with one device or the other. There are some circumstances where I will specifically recommend one particular device. For example, I had a lady come in who had never in her life heard in the high frequencies. In that particular scenario, we made a choice to have an implant that went out way far into the inner ear so that we can stimulate predominantly the low frequency areas. Cochlear implants in general stimulate the mid to high frequencies of the inner ear and don't reach the real low frequency areas. If the high frequencies are not going to be used because the inner ear doesn't have nerve fibers there, then we want an implant that goes deeper in.

Dr. Loren Bartels: There are a few scenarios where we will make a specific choice. Most of the time though, we want the patient to go through the device selection process and make their own decision. There are some other things that come into play. There are people who need MRI scans on a recurring basis. All three of the major companies are nominally MRI compatible, but the most compatible with MRI right now is the new Advanced Bionics device that's been out about a year. With that particular device, you can have your head in any position in an MRI machine and not have a problem. With the other two devices, you have to be careful to go into the MRI machine nose up. Now, almost all MRIs are done nose up, so it's not very common with any of the devices to have a problem with MRI machine with the current devices. But there are a few scenarios where Advanced Bionics would be better.

Richard: What about the array that goes into the cochlea? Does that make a difference and when you make a choice?

Dr. Loren Bartels: Well, it turns out that all the company's dominant arrays now are about 23 to 24 millimeters long. Advanced Bionics has 16 electrodes in that distance. Cochlear Corporation has 22 electrodes, and then MED-EL for their 24 millimeter electrode has 12 pairs of electrodes. In terms of depth of insertion, they're going to be pretty close. There is a longer device with MED-EL that's 28 millimeters long and another one that's 31 millimeters long, but the vast majority of people are going to get the same depth of insertion regardless of which device they pick.

Richard: But you just mentioned before that you've done studies recently here that there was not much difference between the results of all three brands.

Dr. Loren Bartels: That's correct. There is a study that was done a number of years ago in Hanover, Germany that compared the three brands and Advanced Bionics and MED-EL were statistically equal with Cochlear Corporation, them not being as good, but Cochlear Corporation has done a lot of software work in the interim, and in our study of the last number of years, we think the hearing benefit is the same among the three devices.

303

Richard: Now, my next question to you is, are there times to advise a candidate not to proceed with the cochlear implant? What would those be?

Dr. Loren Bartels: Well, there are a variety of scenarios. The first thing to mention is that the insurance rule and the Medicare rule is we have to prove with a best possible hearing aid set up that they won't do better than certain criteria with hearing aids than with a cochlear implant. And those criteria are based on the fact that you have to meet those criteria in order for you to perceive a cochlear implant to be better than a hearing aid. They first have to meet those criteria.

Dr. Loren Bartels: Now, those criteria are a little fuzzy. There are some scenarios where one ear has hearing aid usable hearing and you can put a cochlear implant in the other ear. There is some fuzziness in those criteria that we can work with. For example, I saw a lady yesterday from Miami who had been tested and said she was a cochlear implant candidate down there. But when we put her through testing here with our hearing aids, she was not a cochlear implant candidate. And the problem was, she was tested with hearing aids that were not best possible. One of the challenges we have, make sure that we test them with the best possible hearing aid fitting. You don't want to subject somebody to surgery that you can really reach with hearing aids well enough.

Dr. Loren Bartels: There are a few other scenarios that are unique. For example, I had a man a number of months ago who had Meniere's disease. It was really bad in one hear, so he was having recurring bad vertigo spells in an ear with very poor hearing. He had a moderate hearing loss in the other ear. We had done all the conservative things. The next step was to drill out his balance organ in surgery. And if we do that, then we may lose the ability to put a cochlear implant in later. We sought permission from his insurance company to put a cochlear implant in that ear at the same time we drilled out the balance organ. We drilled out to balance organ, but we kept the hearing organ and put a cochlear implant in and he's doing very

304

well. And that's called a cochlear implant with single-sided deafness, and there is now a growing body of research that a cochlear implant often helps in single-sided deafness.

Dr. Loren Bartels: So, there are a variety of scenarios. There are some scenarios that we can't help. An example would be a gentleman I saw who had a skull fracture and both of his inner ears were broken, cracked, and had turned to solid bone. Well, I can't get cochlear implants into ears like that that are likely to work. There are some scenarios where you can't get it in. I saw a gentleman last week who had had surgery 40 years ago in his left ear. That ear went deaf. He's had some surgery in his right ear. He's got moderate to severe hearing loss in the right ear. He wanted to know if a cochlear implant would work in his left ear. Well, as a complication of the surgery he had 40 some years ago, that left inner ear has turned to a bone. There's no fluid space, no nerve fibers I can put a cochlear implant in.

Dr. Loren Bartels: There are some scenarios where I can't get in. Part of being a candidate is I have to make sure the anatomy will accept the cochlear implant, and then part of it is you have to be bad enough and we have to do that with appropriately fitted hearing aids. We have to test you with the best possible hearing aids.

Richard: That's a question I hear all the time from new inquirers about it, so that's very helpful information. Vestibular issues, balance issues, do you see those all the time?

Dr. Loren Bartels: We do see people with things like bad Meniere's disease in both ears. They have episodes of bad vertigo in both ears and then get progressively worse hearing. And some of those people become cochlear implant candidates. In fact, some of them get cochlear implants in both years, so there are vestibular issues at times. There are times when a vestibular issue will guide us to do one ear instead of the other. One of the possible side effects of cochlear implant surgery is dizziness. If a person has a real bad balance organ in one ear and both ears are candidates for a cochlear implant, we might choose to put the implant in the ear that has poor balance so that we don't risk injuring the balance and the better balance organ ear.

Richard: Do you have some kind of idea of percentage of people that might come into that category?

Dr. Loren Bartels: Well, let me just in general say a rough number. About 10% of cochlear implant candidates have major balance issues that we have to deal with as part of the decision process.

Richard: What about tinnitus? Does that get alleviated with a cochlear implant? Do you see that?

Dr. Loren Bartels: About 60 to 70% of people who have tinnitus and meet cochlear implant criteria have less tinnitus when the cochlear implant is turned on. Tinnitus by itself is not a reason to do a cochlear implant except on very rare occasions. But in general, a person with troublesome tinnitus does better with a cochlear implant turned on.

Richard: And after the candidate decides on surgery, about how long is the average period until they get it?

Dr. Loren Bartels: Usually just two to four weeks.

Richard: And when you do surgery ... They ask me this all the time. I say it's an out- patient procedure but I was put under when they didn't mind mine, so I have no clue how long it takes. What's your-

Dr. Loren Bartels: Well, the surgery itself takes about 45 to 55 minutes under general anesthesia. The total anesthesia time is about an hour, and it is done as an outpatient with rare exceptions.

Richard: And the follow up visits with you?

Dr. Loren Bartels: We see them back at two weeks and that's when we also start doing the cochlear implant tune up.

Richard: Okay. Now my next question is about your relationship with audiologists. What is your relationship with them?

Dr. Loren Bartels: Well, we have an integrated practice here, so we have seven audiologists and three ear doctors, and we just work closely together. And when we have challenges for making decisions on cochlear implant patients, we talk to each other to see where we ought to go.

Richard: Okay. I know that my next question to you was about your greatest success stories and your most difficult cases, and I also understand you recently did a five month old child, which is astounding to most people when I say that. Could you talk a little bit about that?

Dr. Loren Bartels: Well, one of the questions that's critically important is at what age for a baby does it become less likely that they will have normal speech and language. The statistics show that if you don't get the cochlear implant in before six months, there will be some permanent language deficit. In Poland, which is a place that does the most pediatric implants in the world, they do them now down to four months of age. How young am I willing to go is a good question.

Dr. Loren Bartels: This five-month-old baby is a baby who has a genetic abnormality called Connexin 26. With a Connexin 26, we know this baby is never going to hear without a cochlear implant. And then the question is, when is the baby big enough and mature enough to tolerate anesthesia? Lung maturity in children reaches suitable age somewhere in the four to eight months of age. A premature baby or a sickly baby will take longer to become healthy from a lung perspective. This particular baby was relatively large, so at four and a half months, that baby weighed already 17 pounds and the baby's head was plenty large enough for a cochlear implant, so we were willing to go ahead early on this baby.

307

Dr. Loren Bartels: That's one of those things where we saw this child when the baby was about six weeks old. The child failed infant hearing screening. All babies born in birth facilities, hospitals or birth centers are required by law to have their hearing checked. That's called infant hearing screening. The baby failed. That was repeated. Something called auditory brainstem responses testing was completed. Otoacoustic emissions testing was completed, and the baby turned out to be deaf. And then on an urgent basis, I asked the geneticist to see the baby and the genetic testing was done. The testing proved that the baby was never going to hear.

Dr. Loren Bartels: Then the question was, how soon can we get the implants in? Well, since six months of age is when you start losing something on a permanent side for speech and language, we want to do the baby as soon as we can after the baby's healthy enough. We just made plans to see the baby regularly until I felt the baby was large enough and made sure the baby looked healthy, breathing well, functioning well. This baby was a relatively large baby, so we were happy to go ahead at five months. I probably would've done this baby at four and a half, maybe four months because it's just a big baby. There are other babies where I wouldn't make that choice.

Richard: It's interesting because I see this on social media time after time from parents with very young children concerned about the bulging of the implant, the appearance of the child, how the child's going to do in society with the cochlear implant, because obviously it's a very traumatic experience for a parent. Your experience with the appearance is?

Dr. Loren Bartels: What we do is partially recess the implant in bone. The child skulls are not as thick as adult skulls, so we can't get it in as far. But by and large, when people realize what a huge difference a cochlear implant in a baby makes, the fact that you've got something relatively large appearing for a baby on the side of the head isn't really an emotional obstacle. If you consider what happens to people who grow up deaf in terms of language development, cognitive development, and emotional issues versus those who get implants, it's a no brainer.

Richard: Now, you've been with cochlear implants from the beginning. What do you see the future, robotics, or something changing you can see in the future?

Dr. Loren Bartels: At present, we think cochlear implants are going to become better in terms of reliability of electronics and I think ability to use microphones to optimize hearing and noise will improve. Something we hope happens eventually is that some of these disorders where the inner ear gets progressively worse, we will learn how to fix with genetics. There may come a day when we can send new genetic material into the inner ear and make the inner ear rebuilt. That's not anytime soon, but that's really the long term hope.

Richard: What about the preservation of residual hearing? Again, that's a topic I hear time after time.

Dr. Loren Bartels: There are candidates, and about 80% of the time, we can save at least some hearing and the operated ear enough to use a hybrid cochlear implant system. For example, a man over age 80 with a severe hearing loss is less likely to have hearing salvaged, but by and large, we can save hearing in a good number of ears. Now, it turns out the better the hearing before surgery, the more likely it is we can save some.

Richard: The hybrids. That's become a hot topic. I've seen it again time after time. You mentioned the single-sided deafness, and cochlear implants, again, is a growing field. What do you see about the hybrids?

Dr. Loren Bartels: Well, the hybrid, let me put it this way. The interest in hybrid now has all three companies onboard with FDA approval to do that. There are a little different criterion among the three companies, but in functional terms, if you meet criteria for a hybrid, most places are willing to do that now. There are some animal data that suggests that if you start steroids two days before surgery and continue for two to three weeks after surgery, you're more likely to have hearing preserved. So that's our protocol now is we start steroids two days before and continue them for three weeks after, and it looks like we've got about 80% chance of saving at least some hearing.

Richard: That's a fascinating number. And may I ask about what you would like to see the cochlear implant manufacturers do in the future that will make your job easier?

Dr. Loren Bartels: What they're working on is making it more possible for patients to interface directly over the internet. Part of the challenge for that is that the current insurance and billing pathways don't pay for that. It would be nice to get that all figured out so that people don't have to drive so far for relatively minor things.

Richard: That's true. Again, one of the topics I see all the time, if somebody lives in a place far away from the audiologist, they'll suffer with a poor mapping than drive two or three hours to get there.

Dr. Loren Bartels: Right.

Richard: That would help. Can I ask you, what would you like to add toward candidates considering a cochlear implant?

Dr. Loren Bartels: Well, I mentioned the Bartels kitchen table test earlier. So let me tell you what that is. Fairly simply, you sit across the table from a person with a hearing aid set to whatever is their perception of a best setting. Don't turn any household noise off, and then someone speaks to you with their face covered. If a person talks to you across the kitchen table with their face covered and you struggle to understand, you're probably bad enough for a cochlear implant.

Richard: Or a better hearing aid.

Dr. Loren Bartels: Well, that may be. That sometimes is the challenge is you just need a better hearing aid.

Richard: Thank you so much for your time, Dr. Bartels.

CHAPTER 26 DR. BRUCE GANTZ

LEADING THE WAY TO PRESERVE RESIDUAL HEARING THROUGH ROBOTIC SURGERY AND HYBRID COCHLEAR IMPLANTS.

I first heard the term "Hybrid cochlear implant" when I met David Dorsey (his interview also appears in cochlearimplantbasics.com) in 2017. He had enough residual hearing that he was investigating these devices.

A hybrid, as the name implies, combines a cochlear implant to assist those missing frequencies along with a hearing aid to help the natural acoustical ones.

It was David who mentioned Dr. Bruce Gantz as the expert in hybrid cochlear implants and he was willing to travel from Florida to Iowa for the surgery.

I interviewed him not long after his activation in 2019. In 2021 he returned to Dr. Gantz to receive his second hybrid for his other ear.

Dr. Gantz has been in the field of cochlear implants for four decades. All the way from the pre-FDA approval days to the most recent advancement, robotic cochlear implant surgery. He explains why robotic surgery the key to better retention of residual hearing is.

Dr. Gantz took time from his busy schedule to sit down with me to talk about the history of his involvement with cochlear implants, his specialty and the exciting development of robotic surgery and his vision of the future.

Richard: Good morning. We are talking this morning to Dr. Bruce Gantz, and I'd like to start if you give me your name, the date, and the city that you're in.

Dr. Bruce Gantz: My name is Bruce Gantz. This is November 16th, 2021.

Richard: And what city are you speaking from?

Dr. Bruce Gantz: I'm in Iowa City, Iowa at the University of Iowa.

Richard: Terrific. I'm so glad you sat down to talk with me this morning because I have a lot of questions about hybrids. Give me a little bit of background how you got into the field and where you are today?

Dr. Bruce Gantz: I've been practicing for over 40 years. Originally when I went to medical school, I was interested in cranial facial surgery and cleft palates, and I thought that's something that was very interesting, and it led me to otolaryngology. And lo and behold, I found out that the ear and neuro-otology was much more exciting than dealing with patients with plastic surgery issues. I've been fortunate throughout my career to train at outstanding institutions. The University of Iowa and Dr. Brian McCabe was an outstanding otologist, neuro-otologist. And then I was able to train in Switzerland with Professor Ugo Fisch at the University of Zurich, who was an extremely innovative skull-based surgeon. And that's where I really started to explore cochlear implants more.

Dr. Bruce Gantz: During my residency, I was sent to Bill House by Dr. McCabe to learn how to put in a single channel cochlear implant. And I spent two weeks in Los Angeles meeting with Bill and Derald Brackmann, and several the other people, and Laurie Eisenberg and people that were involved in the cochlear implant team at that time. This was in 1979. We put in our first cochlear implant at the University of Iowa in 1980, in the spring of 1980.

Richard: Was it FDA approved at that time? Or you were on the outside of it?

Dr. Bruce Gantz: That was on the outside of the FDA. The FDA did not have a lot of control of implants at the time. And I can tell you about an experience bringing back implants in my suitcase from Europe, in which the FDA, they really weren't that interested in implants at that time. It was really a group of individuals in different centers that were really developing cochlear implants. And I learned in Europe about the Vienna implant, which became MED-EL. I met Ingeborg and Erwin Hochmair in 1982. And I met Kurt Burian who is the surgeon that put the devices in, and I watched him do that. I went to Paris, and I met Chouard and watched him place different electrodes in cochleas drilling individual holes, and then saw these patients. I met Bonfi who was another surgeon in Europe, Douek in London.

Dr. Bruce Gantz: So, I had quite an exposure to different individuals. And I learned that we were not going to build a new implant in Iowa. But one of the opportunities at the time were to do some uniform measurements of outcomes in these patients. And that's how we evolved as a center where we developed some testing strategies with Dr. Richard Tyler, who is the audiologist at the time with us, and we developed the Iowa protocol. And we then started to apply for research money through the NIH. The first time that we applied, we were summarily dismissed. We learned a lot about grantsmanship, and they brought me onto a committee in the Neurology Institute to look at clinical trials. And we then developed a system that we have been able to continue to parlay through seven five-year cycles over the past 36 years. That is how I have gotten involved with cochlear implants.

Richard:

Your cycles of grants obviously led to advancements in every step of the way. And I think what the listeners are interested in right now is how you got involved in the hybrid cochlear implant. If you could explain that to us and how you got involved in that.

Dr. Bruce Gantz: Well early on, we were only implanting individuals that were so profoundly deaf that they couldn't even hear themselves talk. Many of them had been deaf for 40 to 50 years.

Richard: That would be me. That would be me.

Dr. Bruce Gantz: Yes. And we started exploring different criteria. A group of us felt that individuals that had more residual hearing and less duration of deafness, which was one of the issues that we were exploring at the time, did better. We started thinking about ways in which we could potentially expand the criteria to people with a little more residual hearing. At the same time, I had become involved with Graeme Clark's group in Australia and Cochlear Corporation. We were the first people to put in a multi-channel cochlear implant in the United States outside of Melbourne, Australia in 1983. That was almost 40 years ago. We've had a good collaboration with them over the years. And I brought this concept to them to explore. And we designed an electrode in 1998 in which it was going to be shorter because my objective was to try and do as least damage as we could in the inner ear. And I knew that Bill House and his team had used single channel implants in a few patients to suppress tinnitus.

Dr. Bruce Gantz: They were able to do that in some patient and they preserved some residual hearing. These were not deaf patients at the time. I thought originally that we would use a six-millimeter implant just like Bill House, multi-channel. We designed it with six channels, and we got FDA approval in 1999 to implant the patients. We implanted three patients with a six-millimeter device, and we learned some very interesting things. We were able to preserve residual hearing in all three. We were able to preserve not only their level of identification of pure tones, but we were able to preserve their residual acoustic discrimination. And so that was really an eye-opening experience for us. It's better to be lucky than good, right? And we turned these patients on. And what we found was that it was very high frequency because it was very much in the first few millimeters of the cochleas, and these patients got some benefit out of it.

Dr. Bruce Gantz: But they were disturbed about the high frequency pitch that they were perceiving in this area, because we were probably at 20K to maybe 8K in the area that we were stimulating. So, we went ahead and stopped that. And we got permission to go with a longer device and we went 10 millimeters, and we put the electrodes a little bit more apical so that we got past this first four to six millimeters of very high frequency area. And fortunately, we did well with that device. The S8 was a device that was the first hybrid that we used in a clinical trial of about 80 patients over a long period of time. And I can tell you that I still have some of those patients that were implanted in 2000. It was in 2000 that we implanted the 10millimeter device that still have residual acoustic hearing today 20 years later. The idea evolved out of that experience. We were not the first to publish this data.

Dr. Bruce Gantz: We did not publish our first three cases because we wanted to wait and see what happened. Unfortunately, there was someone else in Europe that published one single patient that beat us to it. But that's life. Anyway, we have continued to explore acoustic plus electrical processing. What we identified with these patients early on was the fact that when you preserve that low frequency hearing, the real advantage was that you improved your hearing in noise, because what that low frequency did was allowed the listener to discriminate the vocal cord vibration or the fundamental frequency from the surrounding noise. And with electrical processing, we can't do that very well.

Richard: I have a question for you right now. You were looking at candidates, how much residual hearing did they have? Is there a percentage wise basis that you decided to do the hybrid?

Dr. Bruce Gantz: At the time, we were looking at people that had low frequency hearing around 60 decibels in the lows, 125, 250 and 500. And above that, they could be profound, 80+ Db. We found out that we could preserve acoustic discrimination by not going very far into the cochlear. There were two other advantages. So that first is hearing better in noise. And our patient populations are much better in acoustic plus electric than they are electric only in hearing in noise. And they also get the perception of melody and music because of the low frequency information that is still there. And so that was a real advantage to our patients, so they could hear music and appreciate melody. The third advantage was that if you preserved residual hearing in both ears in the low frequency, your spatial hearing where your localization was preserved, we found out early on in our experimental work with binaural implants that people that have two implants can tell where a sound is coming from.

Dr. Bruce Gantz: Whereas if you have one implant and some residual hearing acoustically on the other ear, you have no spatial orientation. And that was an eye opener to us that if you preserve low frequency in both ears, then they had spatial orientation again, that they could localize sound. So those were the three real advantages of preserving low frequency hearing. Unfortunately, our electrical processing algorithms in all our cochlear implants do not provide that low frequency fine structure that is important to hearing the differences in noise and melody. And we've never been able to develop algorithms that can do that. Now, we have a few people that are real stars that use cochlear implants with electrical processing and can experience music and understand music. I have a woman who was a piano teacher, and she judges piano competitions with a cochlear implant in place, which blows me away.

Dr. Bruce Gantz: But it's possible in some patients. So that's how we got involved with the hybrids, and we are continuing to explore that. We know that it takes time for people with acoustic plus electric hearing to get that centrally and fuse that information that initially when they're programmed, they do not like it. And because of that reason, we have many audiologists and people in the implant world that don't believe that this is very worthwhile. But I can tell you-

Richard: That misconception is something I fight all the time. That's a number one issue of a misconception that keeps people on the fence. It annoys the hell out of me.

Dr. Bruce Gantz: So unfortunately, once you put an implant in that destroys the residual hearing, you're not going to ever get that back. And so, we must develop strategies that are better at preserving low frequency. I can tell you that our 10-millimeter devices are the best. We have about 75 to 80% preservation of acoustic discrimination with those shorter devices. The longer devices are not quite as good.

Richard: I have a question at this point, the first three you implanted with the very short device that were annoyed by the high frequency, did you re-implant those people? Or do they just live with it?

Dr. Bruce Gantz: No, we did explant two of them with standard devices, because we didn't know if we could keep the residual acoustic hearing.

Richard: Part two of my question is this, you're talking of the length of the electro array. Now, some of the companies claim they have the longest array possible, and people are confused sometimes if the longer array helps them better with discrimination or just the overall experience. Is there something in the longest array that helps? I understand, yes, probably not going to preserve residual hearing if you go that long. What's your experience in that area?

Dr. Bruce Gantz: I will tell you that the brain has the capability of transferring frequency information so that we can accommodate to the place pitch, okay? And the cochlear is tuned like a piano. The highs are in one area, the lows are in the other. And we know that if you want to get better pitch matching initially, if you put a longer electrode in, the patient will be more satisfied. And I will tell you that when we are doing patients with single-sided deafness and they have normal hearing in one ear and you put the implant in the other ear, we found that a longer electrode allows them to adapt more quickly, okay? Now, we also know that in the patients with shorter arrays that are preserving residual hearing that you can adapt to the place pitch offset of up to four octaves. You can transfer that over time. But it's not immediate. It may take six months to a year to get that transposition.

Dr. Bruce Gantz: But the brain can learn that there's new regions being stimulated with higher frequency that can be perceived as low frequency. You can put the low frequency information in a high frequency area and the brain will then accommodate to it. But it doesn't happen overnight. And that's part of the issue with the hybrid implants in patients that they must know that they must accommodate to this place pitch shift. And it takes a little bit of time. But once you get it, it's very beneficial.

Richard: Is there a special rehab patients must do?

Dr. Bruce Gantz: We send them home with some recordings to listen to. We have them listen through their implant only for periods of time during the day to help reorganize this information. But it takes time and individuals differ on how much time it takes. And it probably has something to do with their cognitive function. We all don't learn at the same rates and that's part of the variability and performance of all these devices. We have some stars in every device and we have some failures. Or not failures, but not as good in every device.

Richard: Okay, let's not talk about failures here.

Dr. Bruce Gantz: No.

Richard: I have reminded people that there are no guarantees in life, but the vast, vast, vast majority of cochlear implant recipients get optimal results, but life does not have any guarantees.

Dr. Bruce Gantz: You're exactly right.

Richard: I'd like to ask you, a candidate comes to you, you're doing the qualification to see if they're a candidate. And I believe from my experience of talking to hundreds of candidates, when the word hybrid comes up, I say, "I don't know how they qualify you for that." Do you ever discourage somebody from going along with the hybrid? Can you talk about the qualification process?

Dr. Bruce Gantz: Sure, okay. We know that when we put in an implant in the inner ear, we lose about 15 decibels in pure tone thresholds. And it probably has to do with the mechanics of the traveling wave in the inner ear. Some people don't have that as much, some people have more. So, we figured that we want to start with someone that has pretty good low frequency and not somebody that has marginal low frequency. And you must realize that there's another concept we haven't talked about, and that is functional and non-functional acoustic hearing. So, this concept evolves out of the fact that when you amplify acoustically, there are certain limits that the ear has. And somebody that has about 85 decibels of low frequency hearing in the 125, 250 and 500, if you amplify them as much as you can amplify them with a hearing aid, they're not going to get any information. So that functional ability, it's better if you have somebody at above 80 decibels with their residual hearing.

Dr. Bruce Gantz: So, we want to start with people better than 55 decibels in the low frequencies. If we lose 10 to 15 Db, you're down to maybe 70, and we can amplify 70 with an acoustic hearing aid. If you don't have that, then we discourage using the hybrid because we've tried it in people between 55 and 80 and we find that we can't amplify acoustically if we don't have the drivers to use that residual acoustic hearing. So that's how we would help make that decision.

Richard: Some surgeons leave it to the candidate to choose which company based on the implant array. How do you choose the array you're using with the patients because people ask about that all the time?

Dr. Bruce Gantz: Well, I will tell you that three companies that are out there right now provide a pretty good product. I mean there have been missteps by all three companies. They had issues and recently the latest issue has come with Oticon, which just trying to get started in the United States. And they had a recall. But every one of the companies, Advanced Bionics, Cochlear Corporation, or the Nucleus device, and MED-EL have all had issues over time. So, in fact, if you have a standard cochlear implant patient, you're not trying to do anything special and you're not concerned about preserving residual hearing or something like that. All three devices provide an average improvement in word understanding to around 50% word understanding, 50 to 60% word understanding, with an electrical only a processing.

Dr. Bruce Gantz: When we are talking about hybrid or preserving residual hearing, sometimes we are asking patients to participate in certain research projects that we do. And one company may have a device or a design that we are more interested in exploring questions, and we will ask them if they would participate in this research. And so, I will tell you that right now, you toss a coin in the air as to the reliability of these devices now in the longstanding lasting of the three companies that are out there. So, I can't tell you that one company is better than the other. Sometimes, the audiologists like the interface and the setting of the device with one company versus the other, and the next company leapfrogs them. And we now are interested in questions about measuring impedance or the amount of current that is being able to be measured through the device and in the cochlea so that we can look at the long-term residual hearing.

Dr. Bruce Gantz: We think that measuring impedance remotely with a patient at home and through their telephone, we might be able to tell them if things are changing in the inner ear that maybe they need to come back to the center and we will try to do some things that might change that. So, there are all questions that we are addressing that may be different than a cochlear implant group that is just putting in cochlear implants that are not asking the research questions that we're asking.

Richard: My question was more not toward the reliability, but about the differences in the ability to hear. What you've answered, the new advancement and remote monitoring is very exciting.

Dr. Bruce Gantz: Yes.

Richard: But I'm most excited about the article I read about you recently of the robotic surgery for cochlear implant. And I'm sure my listeners are going to be hanging onto every word you're about to tell us.

Dr. Bruce Gantz: Marlan Hansen is a faculty member that is now the head of the department. I stepped down as the head of the department in July and Dr. Hansen now became the department head at the University of Iowa Carver College of Medicine. So Marlan and I worked together for the last 20 plus years. He was a resident in our department and then went out to the House group and trained in neurology and came back. And he had another one of our residents who was an engineer and was one of our research residents spending seven years instead of five years in the residence, Chris Kaufmann developed a strategy to implant a cochlear implant at a very slow rate with a motor or a robot. And so, this device is called IOTASoft, the company is iotaMotion. So Marlan Hansen and Chris Kaufmann developed this company as a spinoff because they got a small business administration grant from the NIH to develop the company. And so, they had to develop the company.

Dr. Bruce Gantz: And just in the last month, we got FDA approval for the robot IOTA-Soft. So, we did a clinical trial here with the motor and we implanted, I think it was 15 patients, and we had really good results. We did not try to preserve hearing with these. It was just the concept of safety and efficacy of implanting. This is a disposable robot that is a one-time use. And so, it didn't have to go through the rigors of implantation that the FDA requires of years and years of trials, because we were not implanting anything. And so, the advantages of this robot are that we can place the implant into the cochlear at $1/10^{th}$ of a millimeter per second. You can hardly see it move. And Marlan and Chris Kaufmann did some animal experiments demonstrating that when you are putting the electrode in by hand, it's jerky, even the best surgeons. I've been doing this for a long, long time, and my ability to put the device in very slowly is not as good as the robot.

Dr. Bruce Gantz: What they determined was that when you implant this device slowly, there's less damage to the lining of the inner ear on the inside called the endosteum. And so, the inner ear is protective of the brain and this endosteum layer on the inside of the inner ear, if there's an infection, sometimes it ossifies to protect the brain from an infection getting into the brain because there is a connection between the inner ear in the brain. So, trying to do the least amount of damage to the endosteum is important when you're putting in these devices. We try to put them in slowly, maybe over a 10-minute period. But when you're doing it with a robot and it's just constantly going in there so slowly that you can hardly see it move, it's doing the least amount of damage. And so that's the objective in using the robot. We are about to start now with some patients now that we have FDA approval with some patients that have residual hearing.

Dr. Bruce Gantz: We're hoping that using the robot plus we also have strategies called electrocochleography, which we can measure the activity of the hair cells we're putting in the implant. And we know that if we maintain a certain response that we are probably not touching the basilar membrane and where the hair cells are, and we're probably doing less damage. So, the combination of using the robot with electrocochleography I think is going to help us improve our rates of preservation of low frequency hearing, and I'd like to get to 95% preservation of hearing a year down the line. And I think if we did that, then people would be much more apt to move forward with preservation of hearing.

Richard: I agree with you, and I've just marked it in my calendar interview you a year from now. So, we can do a follow up at that point. Like I said, this is very exciting news. My mission from the beginning is to get people off the fence because less than 5% of the people who could be helped with the cochlear implant move forward. And the preservation of residual hearing is a very important topic. It comes up all the time. So, I'm very excited about that.

Dr. Bruce Gantz: I tell patients and I tell my colleagues and my surgeon colleagues that you only have one chance to preserve this hearing. And if you lose it, then it's a disadvantage for the patient. For the most part, you're going to get an improvement in hearing in quiet, but we need more than that. We don't live in a quiet world. It's hard to watch TV with a hearing aid and it's hard to watch TV with an implant if you don't use closed captioning. Correct?

Richard: I don't watch TV, so I'm- Dr. Bruce Gantz: Okay.

Richard: I'm not the guy to ask. I still prefer reading. Let me ask you again. Now, the future of robotic surgery is everywhere, whether it's joint replacement, heart valves, whatever it is. Where do you see the future of cochlear implant robotics five years down the road?

Dr. Bruce Gantz: I will tell you that we're working on some other potential issues here, and one of the reasons to use the robotic system in the first place was that if we put the implant in 10 or 12 millimeters and a patient lost residual hearing, could we move the electrode more into the cochlear to maybe take advantage of that low frequency region that you were just talking about? And we know that there's a trade off with implanting longer versus shorter. Longer you implant it, the less likely you are likely to save hearing. But could we develop a strategy which we implant the patient maybe 10 or 12 or 14 millimeters. And then if they lose residual hearing, can we advance it? And so that's the concept that we're working on now. And we think we have a strategy that could allow that to be happening.

Dr. Bruce Gantz: We know that if you must open the ear and the mastoid and try and advance the electrode, there's so much scar tissue in the mastoid that it sometimes is difficult to separate the implant from the scar tissue. And so, the company iotaMotion is developing a strategy that you could do this without having to open the ear again.

Richard: This is incredible.

Dr. Bruce Gantz: I think that in the future, we're going to not wait so long to start implanting people. When they have difficulty hearing in noise and they are withdrawing from society, and we know that that can impact cognitive function, why wait for 10 years until they become an implant candidate before you implant them? When we think we might be able to help them earlier, maybe prevent, or I'm not certain that we would ever cure the cognitive decline, but maybe we will postpone it by providing the stimulus of the acoustic information that seems to be so critical for individuals to interact socially. And I think that's where we're going to be going. I think we'll continue to expand the criteria for selection. We will hopefully take people that have less than 50% word understanding and be able to provide them with 80 or 90% word understanding and may be able to hear 70 or 80% of the words in noise. Wouldn't that be nice?

Richard: That would be fantastic. This is one of the most interesting interviews I've done in two years, and I really appreciate your time. Do you have anything you'd like to leave listeners with before we sign off?

Dr. Bruce Gantz: I just think, Richard, that I appreciate what you're doing. We need individuals like you that are supportive of implants and supportive of the technology and supportive of the growth of the technology. And we'll continue to work here at the University of Iowa looking at the interaction between cognitive function and the implant. I will tell you that we are doing some very interesting studies about how words are formed centrally, looking at eye tracking and looking at PET scanning images of tracks of the auditory system. And we know that when you preserve residual hearing, the ability of the brain to recognize the word more quickly occurs much better if you have some acoustic information there than if you just have electrical processing. We know that for a person like you that just has an implant or two implants, you are delayed about 75 milliseconds for each word that you are hearing, because you wait until the word is said instead of trying to recognize the word when each phoneme is said or each syllable.

Dr. Bruce Gantz: Most people with normal hearing can start to recognize the word on the first or second syllable in the word and people with implants wait 75 milliseconds after the start of the word. And what happens then is that the frontal area of the brain, the inferior frontal cortex, becomes more involved in some confusion. And we're not using the areas of the brain in the left temporal area, in the super marginal gyrus that is used to recognize words more quickly. This is the work that we're doing to try and enhance and improve cochlear implants for patients.

Richard: This is fantastic. I really appreciate your time and I'm sure hundreds of our listeners are going to be hanging on to every word like I said at the beginning. So, thank you so much, Dr. Gantz.

Dr. Bruce Gantz: Well, thank you, Richard, for asking me to participate. Glad to help.

CHAPTER 27 DR. HERB SILVERSTEIN

THE WORLD'S LEADING EXPERT IN HYPERACUSIS AND MENIERE'S

For more than four decades, Dr. Herb Silverstein has been a leader in otology and has developed surgical and diagnostic procedures in the area of Meniere's disease and hyperacusis. He is recognized as a world authority and patients come from all corners of the globe to consult with him.

President and Founder of the Florida Ear and Sinus Center in Sarasota Florida, he is also the founder and head of the Ear Research Foundation, which he describes in his interview.

Doctor Silverstein has more honors than space to describe them all. I was privileged to have him take time from his busy schedule to sit down for this interview.

I wanted to cover the basics of Meniere's and hyperacusis and as a bonus within the interview, I learned of his leading role in the trials of FX322, and experimental drug being researched for its efficacy to restore the hair cells within the cochlea. This is a subject close to the heart of many with hearing loss hoping for a cure.

His love of research shines through this interview. That love will keep him going forward for many years to come.

Richard:

This afternoon, we're talking to Herb Silverstein, the world's foremost expert in Ménière's and hyperacusis. Would you just tell me your name?

Doctor Herbert Silverstein: Herbert Silverstein at the Silverstein Institute in Sarasota.

Richard: Can you briefly tell me what Ménière's disease is? Because my own impression is it has a lot of different components, and I'm very confused.

Doctor Herbert Silverstein: It's a disease that involves the inner ear. Most of the patients complain of vertigo attacks, recurrent episodes of dizziness where they're spinning around, nauseated, they throw up. It usually lasts about a half an hour to an hour. And with that, they have some usual problem with their ear hearing. The hearing goes down in the ear and they feel pressure and fullness in the ear and ringing in the ear. So that triad of symptoms of ringing in the ear, hearing loss, and vertigo are what Ménière's disease is.

There are various types of Ménière's disease. That's the classic type. Many times, patients have problem with their hearing part first and they'll have pressure and fullness in their ear and a hearing loss without the dizziness, and they'll come to the doctor with that complaint. A lot of times, the doctor will look in the ear and the ear looks normal, and they won't know what's going on because the patient's just saying that the ear feels funny and it's pressure and it's got ringing in the ears and maybe a little hearing loss. So it can be hard to diagnose when it's early. Fortunately, we have some tests that can diagnose this before it becomes serious with the vertigo attacks and whatnot.

Richard: The question I have is this, if there are components and you go to your general practitioner who has no knowledge of Ménière's, that can cause a long delay in getting the proper diagnosis?

Doctor Herbert Silverstein: The practitioners, they have trouble making the diagnosis. They say the patients complain of dizziness. They'll say, "Go take some meclizine or Antivert and you'll get over it," and they may not go into trying to find out what it is or treat it.

Richard: Well, you mentioned a few minutes ago about if you have a diagnosis, you can do some kind of treatments or to slow it down or whatever. I'm curious about that.

Doctor Herbert Silverstein: We're pioneers in early treatment for Ménière's disease. And I've written some papers called the Subclinical Hydrops, or subclinical Ménière's disease, which is what I was telling about. Just a little pressure in the ear, hearing loss, and some ringing in the ear.

The way we diagnose that is that it's very interesting. We have a tuning fork that at 256, so a C, low C, and we take that tuning fork and we put it near the ear that the patient's complaining of, and we put it on the other ear, and they'll say that they hear the sound at a different pitch. That's the only disease that causes that. When there's too much pressure in the inner ear, they hear the sound at a different pitch than the other ear.

Doctor Herbert Silverstein: Yeah, so that's all you need is that tuning fork. I hold that up when I give lectures and I say, "That's all you need to make a diagnosis of Ménière's disease."

And then what causes Ménière's disease is when we look under the microscope after somebody's passed, we see that the inner ear is swollen, the membranes are all blown out and they're blown out like a balloon. What happens in Ménière's disease, we believe that the pressure builds up in the ear and the fluid builds up in the inner ear. All of a sudden, it ruptures, boom. And there's a mixing of the inner ear fluids and the patients get the vertigo attack and the hearing loss and all this other stuff. And then when it collapses back and starts to heal, the patient feels better, and they start getting back to normal or less symptoms.

Richard: Is there a period of time between the onset and sometimes feeling normal? Is it weeks, months?

Doctor Herbert Silverstein: Actually, with the Ménière's attack, usually after they get over it, after a couple hours, they feel pretty good.

Richard: Then it might come back at any time.

Doctor Herbert Silverstein: Yeah, it comes back. And then it's a very fickle disease. We can't tell whether it's going to come back the next day or next week or next month or a year later. It's very fickle the way it goes.

Richard: Well, some of the people that I've mentored over time, because I'm not a doctor, I'm an interviewer, some of the people I've mentored over time had to give up driving because they just never knew if they were going to have an attack while they were driving. Is that common?

Doctor Herbert Silverstein: Very good comment. This is one of the only times that somebody can drive with dizziness. The reason being is that usually before they get the attack, they get something in the ear, they feel the ear fills out with pressure and they start losing their hearing and there's some noise in the ear and they can pull over to the side and live through the attack. If they can't do that, some patients have a situation where they don't have any warning, they can't drive. But there are not that many that don't know that they're going to get one, get an attack.

Richard: One of your patients that I mentored came from Colorado to see you. My impression was that she hadn't driven for like 11 years. I guess that must have been very rare, severe.

Doctor Herbert Silverstein: Yes. It can scare the person that they don't want to drive. Even if they can tell, they feel that they don't have time to pull over to the side and they don't want to take a chance of having vertigo.

Richard: What are your treatments for somebody who has this?

Doctor Herbert Silverstein: There's a whole bunch of treatments for this. Early on, the treatment is steroids. Low salt diet. We put the patients on a low salt diet. We put them on a diuretic that decreases the fluid pressure in the ear. And there's a drug called betahistine. The betahistine causes increased circulation in the ear and very little side effects, and we treat patients with that.

For the attack of dizziness, we have the patients put Ativan under their tongue, half a milligram. What that does is its sort of like a mild tranquilizer, but it has something to do with the inner ear and it just calms the Ménière's attack down. They may have the attack, but it may be a lot less severe. And if they take two Ativan, it may even be better. They even get less symptoms.

Richard: Is that an off-label use of that drug?

Doctor Herbert Silverstein: Off-label, yeah.

Richard: You've been using that a long time?

Doctor Herbert Silverstein: Right. That, we use instead of meclizine or Antivert, because that, you have to take by mouth, and it takes about 45 minutes to go down. Patients are nauseated a lot of times when they have the attack. With the Ativan, it takes just a couple minutes because it's absorbed into the bloodstream from under the tongue.

Richard: So that's the treatment for Ménière's. What about hyperacusis? Can you explain that, please?

Doctor Herbert Silverstein: Hyperacusis is a strange thing that is becoming more and more common. We all worry about not being able to hear and doing all kinds of things to help the hearing better and whatnot. Cochlear implants and hearing aids and all that stuff. There's a problem that patients have, that some people have where they hear too much. They can have normal hearing or slight hearing loss, and when their sound comes in, it bothers them. It hurts their ear. They can't be near people, they can't go in a restaurant, they can't go to movies, and they become recluse. They stay in the house. They don't want to be talking to anybody because it bothers their ear. The sound of the voice or the sound of the environment just drives them crazy.

Richard: With hyperacusis and somebody who suffers from it, is it a particular sound or is it all sound?

Doctor Herbert Silverstein: That's a good question. There are various types of sensitivity of the inner ears to sound. There's a thing called recruitment. Recruitment is where in patients with Ménière's disease, when they have a hearing loss of, say, 50%, when the sound gets up to 50%, they'll suddenly hear a tremendous increase in the sound in their ear, and it'll bother them tremendously. So that's called recruitment.

And then there's a thing called misophonia, which is they don't like sound, like the chalk on the board where it squeaks. I don't know if you ever remember that when you were a kid. It just bothers you. You don't like that.

And then there's another thing called phonophobia. Phonophobia is fear of sound.

So those things are not something that you can treat with surgery that I developed. But the hyperacusis where the patient is having a problem all the time, various sounds are bothering them and it's changing their lifestyle, the surgery that I developed seems to work very well to help them.

Richard: Could you describe the surgery?

Doctor Herbert Silverstein: Yeah, so it's a very simple operation. It's not very dangerous and the side effects are very minimal. What we do is we take a little bit of tissue from above the ear. The muscle above the ear has a covering called fascia, and we take a little bit of this tissue, and we make little pieces, round pieces of tissue, about two millimeters in size, and then we go lift the eardrum up. We go into the ear while the patient's asleep and we look inside the ear. And a lot of times, we'll find that the little stapes bone, the third bone of hearing, is loose and it's jiggling around in the oval window too much. About half the patients have that. When you touch it, it's very mobile. So we call it hypermobile stapes. So we put a whole bunch of tissue down there on top of the stapes on the footplate and around the stapes, about 10 pieces.

And then the round window, which is the window that moves out when the stapes moves in, that window we cover with some pieces of tissue. What we're doing is dampening the sound waves that are going in. It's like wearing a earplug inside your ear, and it stays there all the time. It seems to work very well, and the patients are able to go into sound and live a normal life again.

Richard: Well, there's no rejection because you're using their own-

Doctor Herbert Silverstein: Own tissue, right. There's no rejection. But sometimes it doesn't work. Sometimes the ears are too hypersensitive. You put the tissue down and it's not enough to dampen the sound waves and the patients will still have the problem. But fortunately, it's not very many of those.

Richard: Is there a future for using computer-generated parts to replace what's loose? Have you looked at that?

Doctor Herbert Silverstein: No. I don't know what that would do. But the problem seems to be more of putting something down there to stop the motion of the ossicles, rather than replace them.

Richard: Well, if somebody has a sensitivity to a sound and certain frequencies, their audiogram will look a little bit strange, a little bit off, right? They would have certain normal hearing and then sensitivity someplace else, or no?

Doctor Herbert Silverstein: No. So what we do is we do what we call a loudness discomfort test. It's called a LDL. We put them in a sound booth, and we increase the sound slowly into their ear and find out what level they can tolerate when it becomes uncomfortable to them. You and I, or normal people, can have 90 to 100 dB of sound and they can stand that. These people, anything below 90, 80, 70, 60, they get upset when they hear sound at that level.

Richard: What about the recovery? You do this surgery, and the recovery for the patients is what?

Doctor Herbert Silverstein: They go on outpatient. They go home the same day. Very little pain. And we take the packing out of the ear in a week, and then they can fly back to wherever they are. And they come in from all over the world for this surgery.

Richard: Where's your furthest patient from?

Doctor Herbert Silverstein: We've done somebody from Ireland recently. Yeah. They come from all over for it.

There's something that we should talk about in the Ménière's, the treatment when the medicines don't work. The treatment is... I invented a thing called the MicroWick, which is a little sponge. My wife used to call it a mouse tampon. Tiny little thing. Well, we would stick that in the ear through the eardrum. What that does is it allows the patients to put the steroids into their ear directly by themselves. The doctor doesn't have to inject it in. And then we treat the patients a month with the steroids. And if you catch the Ménière's disease early, you may abort the whole problem by doing that.

In fact, my wife had that in her only hearing ear. She developed Ménière's disease in her only hearing ear. She had a temporal bone fracture when she was a kid. We gave her steroids in her ear for a week. Fortunately, it brought back her hearing. It cured her Ménière's. Actually, that was the beginning of starting to treat patients with that treatment, because of her hearing loss. She was one of the first patients to treat-

Richard: Using the mouse tampon.

Doctor Herbert Silverstein: Yeah, the mouse-

Richard: Use this. The patient is putting the drug in themselves for an amount of time. And then after a month or so-

Doctor Herbert Silverstein: We take it out. We just pull it out. It doesn't hurt or anything. And we put a little paper patch over it and it heals up. The hole heals up.

Richard: That's amazing.

Doctor Herbert Silverstein: Then the next thing is if that doesn't work, they may still have problems with that. The next thing is a thing called gentamicin, which is an antibiotic that kills the balance center in the inner ear. We put that into the ear. We inject that in and that kills the balance cells, and it will stop the attacks of Ménière's.

Before the gentamicin, the gentamicin has been used for 20, 30 years. Before that, I invented an operation to cure the Ménière's disease vertigo, just the vertigo, by cutting the balance nerve going next to the brain. We go in through behind the ear and we find the nerve of hearing and balance, and we just cut the balance nerve and that stops all the vertigo. You don't see the patient again ever after that. It preserves their hearing, what hearing they have, and it cures the vertigo. We did that from about 1977 to the '90s.

When the gentamicin came out, it was an office procedure. So that was easier to do to the patients than the nerve section, where they had to be in the hospital for a couple days. If the gentamicin doesn't work, we then go back to the nerve section again. So-

Richard: How often do you have to go back and use the alternative?

336

Doctor Herbert Silverstein: The nerve sections we don't do very often. We maybe do three or four a year. But most of the time, the gentamicin seems to work.

Richard: The gentamicin is being used by?

Doctor Herbert Silverstein: By everybody. All over. By everybody. Yeah.

Richard: And if it doesn't work, then they call you.

Doctor Herbert Silverstein: They've learned how to do the nerve section too. They do that too.

Richard: Now my question is this, if it's on one side, you have a balance center on the other, hopefully, you can't cut both.

Doctor Herbert Silverstein: Here's the situation with that. It's usually in one ear, but in 15%, it goes in both ears. You have bilateral. We call that autoimmune inner ear disease when it's in both ears because we think it's related to the immune system that they hit this in both ears.

Dr. Dandy used to, in the '30s, he would cut both balance nerves in both ears. If the patient had a bilateral. What that means, that they have trouble with balance forever. But they walk with a wide-based gait, but they don't have an attack of Ménière's disease. And they have some other symptoms with this when you lose both the stimuli systems. But you can recover from it with therapy. But it's much better to recover from loss of balance nerve on one side than on both sides. If you lose the balance nerve on one side, you're almost normal after a while, after you do therapy and time.

Richard: How much therapy is involved in this?

Doctor Herbert Silverstein: They usually do it for a couple months. And they do the exercises at home, balance exercises at home. Just a couple times a day.

Richard: What's the most important thing a person with Ménière's or hyperacusis should know?

Doctor Herbert Silverstein: Well, that there's treatment for it. We know how to take care of it. And that they need to get it diagnosed and treated, and how severe it is and treated.

Richard: I have four Facebook sites, but one of them is called Hearing Loss, the Emotional Side. This is where people who are totally lost come to find out what's going on, find sympathy, which is what we do. But Ménière's is mentioned so often. I have not really had an opportunity to explain to people. Thank you for your time to do this.

Doctor Herbert Silverstein: Okay. Well, good.

Richard: And if somebody needs treatment, where do they go? Where do you suggest they go?

Doctor Herbert Silverstein: Well, they should go to a center. Somebody specialized in ear work, ear surgery, and ear diseases.

Richard: You advise them to get help?

Doctor Herbert Silverstein: Yeah, definitely.

Richard: I would love to know more about the Ear Research Foundation, what you do, what the objectives are. If you'd take a few minutes to tell us about that.

Doctor Herbert Silverstein: Sure. The foundation, I started in 1979, because I was involved in research all my life and research and development. I felt that research should be part of your practice of medicine, so I started the foundation. Our mission was to do research into finding better treatments for dizziness and for hearing loss, and for also educating the public and educating doctors. That's why we started a training program here, where we have trained 49 doctors now in the procedures that we do, teaching them about Ménière's disease and hyperacusis and all, and many other things that we do with the inner ear.

And then there's community service that we give. We've treated many indigent patients in Sarasota County or in the area where they have a problem with their ears, hearing loss or dizziness. And we've given hearing aids to people that can't afford hearing aids.

It's been a great thing, the foundation, because we've made a lot of discoveries and made a lot of progress and different treatments for hearing loss and dizziness through the years, and we keep on the forefront of research and development. We're one of the top offices for research in the country.

One of the exciting things that we're doing right now, as far as hearing loss, is that we're injecting a medication into the ear that causes regeneration of the little hairs in the inner ear and restores some hearing to patients. We're involved in that and probably have the biggest selection of patients that we're doing that on.

Richard: Is that the RX 322?

Doctor Herbert Silverstein: Yes.

Richard: I had no idea you were doing it here.

Doctor Herbert Silverstein: We're the top office in the country, and we'll be the lead author in the paper that's coming out on it.

Richard: When's the paper expected?

Doctor Herbert Silverstein: We're just terminating or closing down the study now. It usually takes months till they get that done.

Richard: Is this the second or third phase of it?

Doctor Herbert Silverstein: I'm not sure about that. I think it's the third phase. We're going into another phase. We're getting ready to start another series of patients where they increase the concentration of the medication. We're just going to start on that, so that we can get more patients that will have a result from the injection.

Richard: Can you talk about the test at all or that's still under wraps?

Doctor Herbert Silverstein: I can talk about it.

Richard: What about the results that you've seen?

Doctor Herbert Silverstein: Well, I can't talk about that.

Richard: Okay.

Doctor Herbert Silverstein: Yeah, because it's a double-blind study. We don't know the results. We know that some patients have shown improvement, and we don't know who's had the placebo and who's had the real stuff. But we believe that by increasing the dose of the medication, more patients will have a result and have hearing improvement.

Richard: I find it fascinating because I had a progressive loss from scarlet fever, and I had a sudden loss when I was 30. And I did not get a cochlear implant back then because it was very primitive, and I didn't want to lose music and I was waiting for science to find a cure in deafness. I waited 35 years until I got cochlear implants.

So again, one of the most common things I find online discussions are about these tests, that people are waiting to get a cochlear implant until they know what the results of these tests are. They're afraid that if they get a cochlear implant, it will destroy their chances of ever getting something else that comes along.

Doctor Herbert Silverstein: I think that they're trying to do the cochlear implant now and preserve hearing. Try to preserve what hearing is in the ear without destroying it. It's possible that they'd still be able to use the drugs, but I'm not sure about that, because the implant may block the medications going in and whatnot. It's hard to say.

Richard: They might have to remove the implant in order to see if it works.

Doctor Herbert Silverstein: Right. But I'm not sure that-

Richard: Wow.

Doctor Herbert Silverstein: ... they can do that.

Richard: We've covered a lot of ground, and I thank you. Do you have something you would like to add before we close?

Doctor Herbert Silverstein: Just that it's been a great honor and a privilege to be able to help a lot of patients and to come up with a lot of new treatments and different procedures and instruments and things like that that I've done throughout my life. It's been a lot of fun and I'm still working at that advanced age.

Richard: Keep working.

Doctor Herbert Silverstein: I'm going to keep working until the end.

Richard:

I want to live to 140. My work is the budget. I mean, you have the education series coming up. Is that something new that-

Doctor Herbert Silverstein: No, we have that all the time.

Richard: Okay.

Doctor Herbert Silverstein: Yeah.

Richard: I'm going to be promoting the education series on my sites-

Doctor Herbert Silverstein: Good. Great.

Richard: ... and the Facebook sites.

Doctor Herbert Silverstein: Great.

Richard: I've built up an audience. Dr. Silverstein, it has been an absolute pleasure. Thank you so much for your time.

Doctor Herbert Silverstein: All right, Richard. Thank you.

CHAPTER 28 DR. VICKY MOORE

A COCHLEAR IMPLANT AUDIOLOGIST IS YOUR NEW BEST FRIEND FOREVER AFTER YOUR SURGERY

Dr. Vicky Moore is an audiologist and co-owner of The Hearing Spa in Sarasota, Florida. In addition to hearing aids, she does evaluations for cochlear implant candidates, as well as programming for all three major manufacturers. In her interview, she discusses the testing, the cooperation with the surgeon and the manufacturers, and activation from the viewpoint of the audiologist. Her independence gives her a unique perspective in which a new candidate will find enlightening.

Richard: Tell me a little bit about your background, your education.

Dr. Vicky Moore: Initially, I was born and raised in England, and then I moved to the States. When I decided to become an audiologist, at the time the field was going through a transition. So, audiology at that point was a master's degree, and I decided... because I could see kind of the way the future was going... to get my doctorate in audiology, and there were programs opening up with doctoral degrees. I have my doctoral degree in audiology, which is a clinical degree with four years for audiology. I have four year undergrad degree in communication sciences and disorders, so a total of eight years of education to do audiology.

Richard: Why did you decide to go into audiology?

Dr. Vicky Moore: For me it was a little unique. My parents owned a hearing practice, so I kind of worked in the summers, and worked in this field, so that's how I ended up picking audiology. I was born and raised into it, so to speak.

Richard: So okay, you have this practice in Sarasota. How do clients find you? Why do they seek you out?

Dr. Vicky Moore: Most of my patient base comes to me from referrals, people who are having struggles with hearing. We'll also get a lot of referrals from other patients, from physicians, people with all different types of hearing loss. I'm unique, because I work not only with hearing devices, but I also work with cochlear implants and do a lot of testing for other types of services through VA and things like that, so.

Richard: A client comes to you for a hearing aid, and they're struggling. At what point do you say to them, "Let's investigate a cochlear implant."?

Dr. Vicky Moore: When we do a full diagnostic testing, and I do the whole diagnostic testing here, we have a sound booth, and we use the latest equipment, do a full hearing test, and we use something called word recognition. Word recognition is the patient's ability to understand words corrected for their hearing loss. I look at that, and I look at the degree of hearing loss to determine whether a cochlear implant may be the next step. And then if, during counseling, they're open to possibly doing a cochlear implant evaluation when I look at that test result, I explain that this may be the next step. And if they're open to it, we then send them out for cochlear implant evaluation, which is a little different testing.

Richard: The people are very, very interested in what is the evaluation testing for a cochlear implant, so I would hope you would just describe a little bit so that...

Dr. Vicky Moore: Sure. Certainly. The testing for a cochlear implant, we put you back in the booth. It is word testing using sentences, and we use a test called the AZ Bio Test. It was devised by the three main cochlear implant companies, and it's standardized testing for implants. You're doing these words, you're doing them with both hearing aids on, because you have to be amplified and corrected for that test, and then we do right ear only and left ear only. We also do CNC testing, which is another single word set testing, and then we score it, and it's all scored to normative data that the companies put out, and then we look at those scores.

Dr. Vicky Moore: Depending on insurance, there's different requirements for that scoring. For Medicare, typically it's 40% or below, and we can add noise to that. Some of my patients, if their criteria is that they're struggling still, but we know that if we add noise, which will help. We add that noise, and then that's also done with that speech testing.

Richard: Now, there are some of the audiologists I understand do three or four stages of testing. What do you do after that?

Dr. Vicky Moore: After that testing, depending on what we find, if you're a candidate at my practice you'd meet with a surgeon. There's vestibular testing that must be done, so there's balance testing, because we need to find out if one side is better than the other. You must have a CT or MRI, depending on the surgeon that you're seeing, and then follow up with their team to make sure you're a surgical candidate. 'm doing the testing to see if you're a candidate for a hearing device, but there's two parts to it. You can be a candidate on paper, but health wise, if your health cannot sustain a surgery, then you may not be able to have that CI surgery. So that's what we must look at, we have to check all the boxes to make sure that the patient is able to have that surgery.

Richard: Now, how do you determine... because some people go right on to social media, and they say, "I wanted BAHA versus a CI," and they're not clear about the differences. Could you take a few minutes to talk about that?

Dr. Vicky Moore: Commonly, we'll have patients call that will ask for a cochlear implant evaluation. They've never met with a cochlear implant audiologist, some of them have never had their hearing tested, so they're not sure what it is they need. When we do them, we do the initial evaluation, kind of go from there, and talk to what the patient's needs are. Sometimes they just need a hearing device, sometimes they have no hearing in one ear and we can look at a BAHA. BAHA is very good for a patient that has single sided deafness if they have good residual hearing in the other ear. We can do demos of the BAHA, so that's the bone anchored hearing aid, in office.

Dr. Vicky Moore: If we have somebody who meets that requirement, we can do that. Some people don't wish to have surgery, because that is a surgery for that device, so then we look at biCROS or a CROS, depending on what their needs are.

Richard: Talk about the biCROS a little bit, what is that?

Dr. Vicky Moore: The biCROS is a hearing device where you have a hearing aid on one ear, and then a transmitter that looks just like a hearing aid on the other ear. And then we send the sound from the bad ear with the deafness, so to speak, to the good ear. And sometimes on that good ear you must have some amplification, so hence the word biCROS. It's getting some amplification in your good ear-

Richard: From your experience, what kind of percentage of people will the biCROS work for?

Dr. Vicky Moore: We don't see too many people with single sided deafness, but for those that do, our technology with biCROS and CROS devices now has gotten a lot better. I'd probably say about 60, 70% of people will end up going that route, as opposed to getting a BAHA. I think maybe I'm unique, because we don't have a surgeon on site, so my figures may be a little bit skewed because I'm seeing more patients that have either looked at the surgical option, or just don't want surgery, and they know that I do biCROS or CROS hearing devices. They'll come in, but they are successful now with the new technology they have for biCROS and CROS.

Richard: Somebody comes in, and you've tested them, and you've tried to suggest a cochlear implant, do they go into shock, or what's the typical reaction?

Dr. Vicky Moore: That's a good question. Mixed on that one, because sometimes people come in and they have the idea that they may be a candidate for an implant. Sometimes they are completely in shock that they've kind of missed their window for a hearing device, and they're now in candidacy realm for an implant. Not everybody wants to have surgery, some people adamantly won't even consider it because they feel there's a stigma with the cochlear implants, so then you must do what's best for the patient in the limitations of what they'll allow you to do.

Dr. Vicky Moore: I always like to show patients what implants look like, because they're not like they used to be 10, 15 years ago. They're a lot smaller now, we have the Kanso and the Rondo, which is a lot smaller device versus the over the ear. Some people don't like the over the ear options. It's just trying to overcome what their initial objections are, to see if you can figure out why they might not want to go that route. But with an implant, you want a motivated patient, so you never want to push somebody into an implant, even if they are a candidate, because motivation is part of the rehab process. And if they're not motivated, then they may not do as well as we would like.

Richard: It's true that sometimes I've worked with people, it may take a year or two until they finally become motivated because now they're in enough pain of isolation.

Dr. Vicky Moore: That they want to, yeah.

Richard: What about the borderline candidate? The candidate who is maybe...

Dr. Vicky Moore: With a borderline candidate, depending on the hearing loss configuration, there are options. We do have implants that are hybrid implants, which can preserve some of the low frequency, different companies have different names for them, that give you that acoustical component so you're not losing your low frequencies. But we are going in and putting in electrical stimulation in the higher frequencies. We do try to have an open mind on how we can fit patients on what's best for the patient.

Dr. Vicky Moore: A lot of it goes on how long they've been struggling as well, and what their life looks like, social history, what they're doing. I have patients that are younger, that a hybrid would be the way to go, so we want to make sure we preserve as much low frequency information. It depends on the audiogram, patients' motivation, and what they are expecting from life. We always, here, want to make sure that they're aware of all their options. I always say it's my job to make sure you know what your options are. Obviously, it's up to the patient to decide what fits best, but at least they know they didn't leave a facility saying, "I never knew I was a cochlear implant option, and that was never mentioned to me."

Richard: It's funny that you should say that, because many, many people say, "I'm too old for this," or "I've been deaf too long for this," and cochlear implant won't work. And your experience is what?

Dr. Vicky Moore: My experience, that's not true. I have many patients such as yourself, and a few others, which have been pretty much deaf over 30 years, and they're wearing implants and they're doing phenomenal. I call you guys my rockstar patients, so we have our rockstars that are doing so well with implants, and it's kind of, everything in literature that I read when I was in school, and that other people may have seen that talks about how

348

people may not do well with an implant the longer they've been deaf, we're now seeing cases where that is not true. I always tell people give it a chance, because you can't be doing worse than you currently are doing if you are not hearing and you are deaf, so it's definitely a better option than where we are.

Richard: It's interesting that I never met anybody who said, "I'm not doing well, I wish I had never had it done." Have you ever experienced that?

Dr. Vicky Moore: I haven't. We're fortunate at this center, the patients that we see, everybody for the most part does well. We have some exceptions to that rule, but still if I say, "Would you rather go back to where you were?" They wouldn't want to go back to where they were. So even though it's not perfect, it's, the reason you're an implant candidate is because you're not doing well with your hearing aids. So that's why you're in that candidacy criteria.

Richard: Let me ask you another question about candidates that are qualified. Now they must make a choice, and in my case, I have what I call a document dump. You go to the audiologist; they dump the manufacturer's brochures in your lap. Do you help the patient choose, or should that be the patient's choice?

Dr. Vicky Moore: So, a few things that go into that. We work with all three manufacturers, so I like to be able to have access to everything. I have some patients that come in that have done their research beforehand, and they know what they want. Typically, I will advise patients on what is available, what each company's pros and cons are, so to speak. We also look at the anatomy of the ear, because some of them have smaller processors than some of the others. And then the final part of that, in my mind, is up to the surgeon, because they're the one that's putting the electrode in, and different companies have different electrode arrays.

Dr. Vicky Moore: They may think that one may be better for the anatomy of the ear than the other. But I try to kind of give them as much information as I can to make an educated decision.

Richard: But the surgeon does decide for them?

Dr. Vicky Moore: The surgeon sometimes, depending on the anatomy, may say we have to go this route. And they will normally give you a reason. A lot of the time what the patient decides is what the patient gets after we do a discussion. I try to leave it up to the patient to make that decision with as much information as I can get. We have a very active hearing loss association group here in Sarasota, Florida, so I always have people that are potential candidates go to that group. I also try to have them speak to some of my recipients that are working well with the implant, so they can see pros and cons and what they like.

Dr. Vicky Moore: Before they make that decision, it's not something they do lightly. They typically get lots of good information, and weight it out for themselves.

Richard: They understand they can't change the decision once it's implanted.

Dr. Vicky Moore: They do. So that's the one thing that we do make sure, that once you have a manufacturer, and you pick it, that is the manufacturer that you are with. And although we can upgrade the processor, the external piece, the internal piece, that is what you're working with. You have to stick with that manufacturer.

Richard: I'm going to go back to single sided deafness, because that's become a very hot button topic right now, about cochlear implants and single sided deafness. You want to describe how that works? Why would somebody get a cochlear implant for single side?

Dr. Vicky Moore: So, there's research studies that have been done for single sided deafness. I am not a study center, but I have had participants that I have sent to studies. It is something that is recently, like you said, a hot button topic. I have sent people for it, I have not seen it myself with patients, whether they choose to go with single sided for an implant, so I don't know how much I can really speak to that firsthand. But I do know that people are trying it, and it does seem like it is something that maybe the way forward, because we are using better electrodes now, and preserving hearing.

Richard: What about your relationship with the surgeons, and the follow up? What happens there?

Dr. Vicky Moore: We work with two centers. We have a center locally that we work with, I also have a center in Tampa that I work with. Both centers we have full cooperation with, which is nice. Once I find a candidate and I identify him, depending on the candidate they advise me who I would like as a surgeon option, and then depending on what they tell me we kind of go over setting up the appointment with the facility, making sure that we have all the paperwork for them. We set it up.

Dr. Vicky Moore: I do the order forms here in house, and then we send them to whichever facility they decide to go with. And then after that, once they've had their surgery, they do a preop first visit, a preop visit, surgery, and then a postop, and then they're back to me and I see them for the remainder of their care. And then they may see their surgeon annually, or every two years depending on what the surgeon decides. I take over care from there, and then send reports to the surgeons.

Richard: What about your relationship with the manufacturers? Do they provide support for you, or training?

Dr. Vicky Moore: They do. For us to be a certified center, which means we must have support from the manufacturers. As I said, I work with

Advanced Bionics, Cochlear, and MedEl, and all of them we have good relationships with their representatives. I meet with them at least once every quarter, and they give me their updates, I attend their trainings. If we have a software update that gets sent to us, and we make sure that patients then get that update if needed. It's definitely a very good relationship, a close relationship with those manufacturers, because we want to make sure that if there's an update or a recall or something, that we know about it.

Richard: Well, do talk about the training you get from them, because I think that candidates would be interested in what kind of training do you get from the manufacturers?

Dr. Vicky Moore: A lot of the manufacturers provide continuing education units, so we call them CEUs. I would say once a quarter, again, they're holding an event that we attend to. Either locally, or I have gone to Atlanta, and Colorado, for different events to get training. Whenever a new product comes out, or if they introduce an upgrade, or something like that, they always provide a training, which we go to. And then we do a one day training, or two days, depending on how significant that upgrade is.

Dr. Vicky Moore: They'll also come in office and do trainings, so I need training and can't make a training in a different state, they will come in and have representatives who train us. Once we get trained, we get certificates to say that we've been trained. When I started doing implants, I'm going back a little bit here, they used to do an online course, which you could complete, and they had different modules before they would allow you to start taking on CI patients. I have my practicum courses, which I did when I was in school. I also worked with a CI audiologist for a year when I was a graduate student, and then I also passed those practicum courses and modules through the manufacturers, to make sure that I was able to see CI patients.

Richard: Let's talk about when things go wrong.

Dr. Vicky Moore: Things never go wrong.

Richard: Things... Okay.

Dr. Vicky Moore: Optimistic.

Richard: Okay. Things do go wrong, people are always worried about that, so if you have a recipient who's saying, "I'm not hearing very well, blah blah blah..."

Dr. Vicky Moore: So occasionally, things will go wrong. Occasionally, there are times when... thankfully it does not happen very often... but we could have a failure. A failure in my world is when everything is working with the processor, everything is connected, software looks good, we're still not getting sound. So sometimes that means internally, the electrode just stopped working. And as I said, thankfully, I've been doing these 12 years, and I see probably over 100 CI patients, and we've only had one. So, I have been very fortunate. And that was a known recall by one company. When all else fails, you have a failure, we bring out the team, because we have a closer relationship with the team. They must do what we call an integrity check, to check the integrity of the electrode-

Richard: Your team is from the manufacturer.

Dr. Vicky Moore: The team is from the manufacturer, they check everything, and that's when we determine what is going on. And then at that point, we have to make a decision from there. Sometimes it's typically a re-surgery type situation.

Richard: From the audiologist's point of view, activation day, people go online, social media, and they see all these happy faces being activated. What's your experience as an audiologist? Talk about activation day.

Dr. Vicky Moore: So, activation day has changed due to social media, I will say that. Expectations are definitely very high now with activation, and we also hope and pray that an activation will go that way, but most of the time, realistically when we do an activation, you will hear some sounds. Typically, I've been told I sound like Mickey Mouse, Donald Duck, the whole gamut. But you don't hear speech straight away like you normally did, it's not something that sounds normal, natural, like you remember. It takes the brain a while.

Dr. Vicky Moore: So occasionally we'll find somebody who can hear straight away when we activate them, but that is very, very rare. I know online when they do the activation it seems like everything, they just start hearing straightaway, which is not the case. And we normally set things softer, so we typically work through what we call progressive MAPs. I call it my baby step approach. We don't turn things up to where they should be straightaway. We start a little softer and then progressively work up to the MAP that we need, and that is what we call the processing strategy we put in the processor.

Dr. Vicky Moore: We do a little bit at a time, and counsel a patient week one you want to be on your lower MAP, and then turn it up a little bit to your second and third and fourth. There is a little more to it than just switching it on, and then being able to hear straightaway. The brain must get used to the stimulation, and that most of the time takes a while. It's not an instant thing.

Richard: How many return visits do they need after they have activation?

Dr. Vicky Moore: My protocol for visits is we see you for activation, then we typically see you about two weeks later. Then I will see you in another two weeks, then depending on how we're doing, we will see you at about two months, and then three months, and then every six months after that. But some of that does vary depending on my patient. Somebody who is doing well, we may not see them as much. But somebody who needs a little extra help, then I may see them more, so we do have that flexibility built in if needed.

Richard: And what about your greatest success stories? What do you have?

Dr. Vicky Moore: I'm talking to one of my greatest success stories right now, you know. Richard is right here. Sometimes you just get a patient that, even though you think on paper may not do as well as you think they will, they do phenomenal, and Richard, I'm sure, won't mind me sharing that he scores over 80% on his AZ Bios with his implants. Prior to that we were at zero, so definitely huge improvement. I have a few more patients, similar situation, who have been deaf for a long time and now wear implants, and now can function and hear close to as normal as I think we can get with the implants in everyday life.

Dr. Vicky Moore: So that's one of the reasons why I do this job, is because I know that for every patient, although everybody is different, we can get them hearing better, and I know what an impact it is to hear on their lives, so they can hear again.

Richard: Talk about your most disappointing activation?

Dr. Vicky Moore: I had a patient who, and I think some of this does come down to motivation, just was not motivated. Her family wanted that implant to be done, and we did it purely because her family wanted it to be done, but I think her heart wasn't in it. It was sad, because from the get-go, the sounds were not appreciated, she didn't like what she heard, and then trying to get somebody to wear something when they don't like the way it is and have a hard time looking at the future. Because with implants, it's not an overnight, it's a long-term goal.

Dr. Vicky Moore: We always say, you'll be doing better in about six months. Six months is a long time to wait when you're eager to hear, and so we could not get that person to wear it for the six months to just commit to the rehab. And in the end, they ended up taking it off at around three, four months, and unfortunately, even though the family was heavily motivated, the patient was not motivated.

Richard: She wasn't.

Dr. Vicky Moore: We just can't do it.

Richard: Are there features you would like to see the manufacturers add to Cis?

Dr. Vicky Moore: Definitely. I would like to see more of the Bluetooth improvements. We have it in hearing aids, where you can use the hearing aid as your mic, so you don't have to hold your phone up. I would like to see that for implant patients. I'd like for implant patients not to just be committed to one type of cell phone; I'd like them to be able to use an Android as well as an iPhone. I think that should be coming shortly. Automatic features, more with the directional microphones, although we are getting that way. Cochlear has forward focus, we have stereo zoom with AB, but just an improvement on some of the noise reduction. And I do think we're getting there, but just like everything it takes a little bit of time, so.

Richard: I agree with you. Is there anything you'd like to add to the interview, or that new candidates should know from your point of view?

Dr. Vicky Moore: When people come in, if they think they're a candidate, I like them open minded, to listen to what we have to say. Try to always bring somebody with you, because when you don't hear well, four ears are better than two especially when you're not hearing well. Take notes, ask your audiologist any question, there is no stupid question. I think sometimes people don't want to ask because they feel like they should know the answer. There's nothing that you could ask us that we haven't probably heard before, and we'd rather you be knowledgeable and know what you're going in for. So just be your own advocate. Advocate for yourself and your audiologist is there to help you with that every step of the way.

Richard: Thank you so much for time, it's very informative, and I'm sure that new candidates will find a lot of information they can use.

Dr. Vicky Moore: Thank you for having me.

CHAPTER 29 CYNTHIA ROBINSON

THE IMPORTANCE OF SPEECH THERAPY. THE SOONER THE BETTER

Candidates for cochlear implants frequently ask about the need or the role of speech rehabilitation.

Cynthia Robinson, the founder of We Hear Here (wehearhere.org) has more than four decades of experience in the field as an educator teaching deaf and hard of hearing children to listen and talk.

A Phi Beta Kappa graduate from the University of Richmond, she received her master's degree in Deaf Education from the Curry School of Education at the University of Virginia. She was a faculty member and for several years, the Co-Director of the Clarke Schools for Hearing and Speech in Jacksonville Florida.

With her experience as a Listening and Spoken Language Specialist, she is an advocate for mainstreaming children with a hearing loss. She is the author and co-author of several books on the subject as well as the designer of classroom programs to facilitate this objective.

I had the opportunity to ask her to explain why early intervention is important for pediatric cochlear implant candidates and how delay can influence the success of the outcome.

She also offers insights on success of prelingually versus later deafened adults who receive a cochlear implant.

Cynthia elaborates on the role of speech therapy and offers suggestions for finding local sources for speech and language specialists.

Cynthia Robinson: My name is Cynthia Robinson. The date is Friday, August 13th and I am in a very hot St. Augustine, Florida.

Richard: Okay it's hot in Sarasota too. They say people move to Florida for the air conditioner.

Cynthia Robinson: That's right.

Richard: I need to ask a little bit about your background and then I'll go into specific questions.

Cynthia Robinson: Okay.

Richard: Your background is an educator for speech therapists. Tell me a little bit about what that role is.

Cynthia Robinson: My background is in education for the deaf and hard of hearing, and I've been doing it for a very, very long time. Beyond 45 years. I came into the field before cochlear implant technology. I was trained to work with children that could not get full access to sound. Some children benefited from hearing aids and some not so much. 've had two halves to my career. The first half was very remedial and trying to work with children tactically, visually, to produce spoken language. And then the second half of my career was after pediatric implants that I was able to work with people that had access because of the miracle of technology for cochlear implants.

Richard: How do you test if somebody is a candidate for speech therapy? Is there a method you use pre cochlear implants and today?

Cynthia Robinson: I think the most important thing, and I will speak primarily from my perspective as an educator of young children, even though I've had some limited experience with adults, who've gotten cochlear implants, is that what happens when we get cochlear implants is that it's not acoustic hearing, it's not natural hearing. It is a substitute for natural hearing. Typically, once the implants are activated, people will report hearing beeps and clicks initially, then that progresses to sort of robotics speech patterns. And then finally the brain makes a complete adjustment into recognizing speech naturally. And it sounds very natural to the person's ears and sounds very natural when they speak with other people.

Cynthia Robinson: In order to get from beeps and clicks to that wonderful, oh wow. I'm hearing everything very similarly to the way other people hear it. It requires training the brain. By working with someone who's trained to do this process to help the brain acclimate to the signal, you facilitate the progress to really understanding, listening, and spoken language. And depending on the individual and where they were at the time they got implanted, that process may be relatively short, or it may be longer.

Richard: We know that people who get cochlear implants must rehabilitate to get very, very successful results. We understand that. But I was intrigued sometimes when I hear people who've gotten cochlear implants that were pretty lingually deaf, they never really seemed to get to pure speech. Your ideas about that?

Cynthia Robinson: There's actually a very good reason for that. If a child is born, prelingually deaf and that child is identified and the child gets technology with cochlear implants within the first 12 to 18 months, because there is FDA approval starting at, I think it's 10 months now.

Richard: I don't know if it's FDA approved but I know surgeons who have operated at 3 months.

Cynthia Robinson: Okay I don't know any surgeons who've done that. I know a few who've done nine months, but I don't think three is unusual. Anyway, if the children get implanted early, we're looking at the auditory cortex. We're getting the signal from the implant in the cochlea to the auditory nerve and up to the auditory cortex. If you look at the auditory cortex before implantation, you will see nerves running through that auditory cortex, but you will not see nerve bundles. So once the child is implanted, those nerve bundles start to form and what those nerve bundles are, is connections. The brain is connecting and building a robust system that helps us understand and use spoken language and produce it as well, of course, is a big part of it. That is neuroplasticity. It is primarily active between birth and three, it starts to drop off between ages three and five, and by age seven, that neuroplasticity has substantially deteriorated.

Cynthia Robinson: You sort of look at it like a can of Play-Doh. In the beginning, it's very, very pliable. If you leave it out for a while, it becomes stiff. But if you work it hard enough, it's reusable. But if you leave it out over night, when you come back in the morning, it's too hard to do anything with. And I think that's a really good way to understand neuroplasticity.

Cynthia Robinson: If you're looking at an adult who has never heard spoken language and decides to get a cochlear implant, probably, there are always exceptions to every rule, but probably you are never going to help that individual really access true spoken language. They will get detection, they will know that there is sound or not sound, they may get discrimination, which is, oh, I hear a couple of things and they're different. They may even get identification for some things like I hear a siren, I hear a jackhammer, but they may never get to that point of full comprehension of spoken language because the auditory cortex has already given up on forming those connections for sound. And it has moved on because every piece of our brain is valuable. The auditory cortex has moved on to process visual stimulation and tactile stimulation.

Richard: This all makes a lot of sense. And I just must use my own example because I lost most of my hearing while I started having a progressive hearing loss from scarlet fever when I was five. And I wore hearing aids from the age of seven, and I did go to speech therapy for several years. My mom dragged me everywhere, which was fine. I also would address the fact for the story because I do have two pediatric mothers who have interviews with me. And again, when parents find out their children have a hearing loss, there's total panic. What do I do? They deal with the internal conflict. Do I give them a cochlear implant now or let them decide in the future? And I'd like you to address that situation.

Cynthia Robinson: Well, what I tell the parents of young children, number one as a professional, I always have to honor the fact that it's a family's choice, what to do. It is not my choice as a professional to make that decision for them. It's my responsibility as a professional, to provide them with information so that they can make the decision that they feel is right for their child and their family. If a family's goal is for their child to have listening and spoken language, you cannot wait because the neuroplasticity will disappear. You have to decide for that child. You cannot wait for the child to be old enough to make the decision for themselves, or you've missed the opportunity.

Cynthia Robinson: I do work with families who want their children to be bilingual, both in spoken language, French, English, whatever, or bilingual in terms of knowing sign language and spoken English. And what I tell them, if they want to be bilingual for sign language and spoken language, whatever language that is, is that they must address the spoken language first. That the ability to learn sign language, and this is just scientific, the ability to learn, sign language, the brain's ability to do that does not disappear. That option will always be there for them. But if you don't get the implant, when the child is very young, you will lose the possibility to develop listening and spoken language because the Play-Doh will have gotten hard.

Richard: That makes a lot of sense. And I know, I have mentored parents that struggled with that question. And because I mentor people in 24 times zones, I must be very much aware of different cultural aspects of having a cochlear implant. Sometimes it's a little difficult to get them over that hump to say, yes, your child's going to have a cochlear implant that'll stick out. But if they're deaf, it'll be worse. I would like to address adults. You've worked with adults who have gotten cochlear implants and now need speech therapy. How do you determine they need that therapy?

Cynthia Robinson: Any adult who gets a cochlear implant in my professional opinion will need some therapy because they're learning to use that implant. We start at the sound level, and we work up to the word level, and then we work into sentences and phrases. And by then, they've acclimated, and they can understand. Pretty much everybody will need that. If a person has gotten their implant soon after having lost their access to hearing, it's going to be a faster process for them. The longer the person has been away from having hearing, the longer it may take their brain to adjust. But if those nerve bundles are there in the auditory cortex, they will adjust. It's just going to take them time. But if it's the prelingually deaf adult, who has never heard spoken language, yes, they will still benefit from therapy because working at the sound level, they will learn that detection, discrimination, identification. And they may even get to the place that they can recognize some words, but it's going to be a much longer process for them.

Richard: You've just given me food for thought here. Is there a way for the surgeon to see if those nerves have formed before he does surgery?

Cynthia Robinson: I don't know whether there's a way for surgeons specifically to look at that, but it's just a brain scan. It's non-invasive and it's used for research. And that's how we had that information, is that researchers go in, look, and see what is the situation for people who are deaf? What does the auditory cortex look like? And like I say, it's non-invasive and then they look at deaf children. What does it look like? And then they look post-implant, and they look at hearing people. So that's how we have this information about the nerve bundles.

Richard: Is that scan commonly done? Frankly, I've never heard of it before. And I would imagine that somebody who is a candidate, who's worried, is this going to work? What will I get if I got a CI, if they had some information beforehand about their possibility, the chances of success would give them confidence to move forward.

Cynthia Robinson: As far as I know, it's not common in clinical practice, it's more used in a research setting.

Richard: That's fine. I understand. Now, one of the other things I know that cochlear implant recipients who live alone, rehabilitation is tricky. I mean, I've created my own rehabilitation programs, which I share with people to do it on their own. Is any sort of remote rehabilitation available to cochlear implant candidates?

Cynthia Robinson: I don't know about the adult population. Even before COVID, I was involved in a lot of tele practice with families of young children. And of course, once COVID came, everything moved to tele practice. I would suspect that if an adult reached out to a clinic that specialized in working with adult implant users, they would find that tele practice is available, but really COVID has started kind of a new trend. There was a lot of hesitancy about the efficacy of tele practice before COVID, but then there wasn't any choice. And so now I guess, good news, bad news. One of the things that we've been able to gather during this time is how much efficacy is there to doing clinical practice through tele practice alone. And it's turned out to be that it's quite successful. So, I would say that reaching out to a center that you would reach out to in person, but you don't live close to them, or you don't want to travel there, or you're selfisolating because of things that are going on in the community is that reach out to them and just say, I'd like to do this through tele practice.

Richard: I would hope at the end, you can give us a list of sources that people could go to.

Cynthia Robinson: What I can suggest, and I don't really have a list of sources, but what I can tell you is if a person goes to the Alexander Graham Bell website, they can look up people who are certified as listening and spoken language specialist, and they can search for listening and spoken language specialist by state. And it will tell you whether that person's background is speech therapy or education, but everyone listed on the Alexander Graham Bell Academy website is a listening and spoken language specialist. You can find them there.

Richard: That's a terrific piece of information. Would you like to add anything to the people that we're talking to about speech therapy and cochlear implants?

Cynthia Robinson: I think as far as families go, the sooner they have this done, the better off the child is. And I think in terms of adults, having realistic expectations based on what your hearing history is, because we don't want people to go through surgery and be very disappointed. I think helping a person examine their hearing history and the probability that the implant will work for them, in the way that they want, is very important because everyone determines success differently. Some adult users might say I'd just be satisfied if I can hear a big noise around me, if I can just monitor my environment a little bit. Whereas another person might say, I'm not going to be satisfied. Success for me is if it sounds just like I remember the voice sounding or if I can appreciate music. I think looking at everyone's goals along with their hearing history for an adult is probably the most important thing to consider.

Richard: That's fantastic information. I'm sure people are going to benefit tremendously from this interview. I thank you so much for your time.

Cynthia Robinson:

You're so welcome. I'm very honored to be asked.

Chapter 30 Robin Chisholm-Seymour

How to Handle Grieving of a Hearing Loss

Is sudden hearing loss equivalent to an amputation of a limb? Does that loss manifest itself in anger or apathy or something else? Is it different for those who experience a progressive hearing loss versus a collapse of all their hearing?

Recently I posted a question on social media: "Has anyone utilized a grief counselor after experiencing a sudden hearing loss?"

The post resulted in a spate of responses. Some wished they had a resource when it happened to them. Others who found support through family and friends. There were those who "toughed it out" and others who found comfort through the power of prayer.

Robin Chisholm-Seymour, a bilateral cochlear implant recipient, and a fellow member of the Facebook group, Bilateral CI Warrior, has extensive experience in grief counseling for both hearing loss as well as those who have lost their animal companions was gracious enough to sit down with me for an interview to explore this subject.

We discussed grieving in broad and specific terms, common behaviors and coping techniques and commonalities as well as the differences in the way people handle hearing loss.

If you or a loved one has experience hearing loss, Robin's insights will help you find the answers to cope with the loss and find a way forward.

Robin Chisholm-Seymour: My name's Robin Chisholm-Seymour. Yes, it's a mouthful. And it's November 7th, 2021.

Richard: And what city are you in, Robin?

Robin Chisholm-Seymour: I am in Alpharetta, Georgia, which is a suburb of Atlanta.

Richard: Give me a little bit of background about your hearing loss, how old you were. I know you're a bilateral cochlear implant wearer. So just give us a little bit of background about that.

Robin Chisholm-Seymour: Well, my story began, I guess back when I was a child, I was born hearing, but I was around my grandmother who lost her hearing at age 12 from Scarlet fever. She was mainstreamed. She read lips and pretty much did everything. I mean, she was such a role model. And at the time, of course, I didn't know I was going to lose my hearing at all. She never ceased to amaze me how she lived life to the fullest. And what happened in my case, in the early 1980s, I was working in a psychiatric hospital. And at the time they had the overhead speakers for announcing and telling you to do this and that and during a meeting, somebody got up out of the chair and took a phone call. I never heard the overhead page. I decided, and some people suggested, oh, just get your hearing checked.

Robin Chisholm-Seymour: I was in my early thirties at the time. Had my hearing checked. And it had diminished in both ears to the point that I really needed hearing aids. So back in the early 1980s, I started the process of hearing aids and then getting bigger ones and bigger ones and stronger ones, but basically was gradually losing hearing in both ears. And then in 2009, I woke up one morning, I was blow drying my hair and got to this side, couldn't hear the blow dryer. I put it in the other hand, and I didn't have a lot of hearing, but I mean, I could hear the blow dryer and I put it over here. I'm even welling up now. I remember that morning and I just welled up and I thought, oh my gosh. I called my audiologist right away. She said, come right in.

Robin Chisholm-Seymour: She tested me, and I mean, it was all gone. And of course, we don't know why, but both of us cried that morning. We both just kind of let it out and got through with that. And then she said, but I know you've heard about cochlear implants. Honestly, I had heard of them. I didn't know much at all. She gave me a couple names of cochlear implant clinics here in Atlanta and said, go get evaluated. So, I mean, I did that as soon as I could get an appointment, I did not meet criteria the first time. And I was very disappointed, but I was on the cusp, and they said, look, just come back in a few months.

Robin Chisholm-Seymour: I did, I met the criteria and in February 2010, I received my right implant. I wore a hearing aid still in the left ear, but it just continued to diminish. And in January 2012, I got the other ear done. Both ears are now with cochlear implants for about a decade. And I have since then had an upgrade to the processors as well. It's been absolutely amazing for me.

Richard: Okay. Now you have bilateral cochlear implants. What really intrigued me is a question I put up on social media last week, or the week before, asking if anybody had gone through grief counseling, because I think we had a somewhat similar background. The fact that I had a progressive loss and a total collapse in my hearing in one month when I was 30 and I went into a tailspin and eventually I got therapy. The theme of this interview is about grief counseling. And I understand you have a lot of experience. I would like to go right into that topic about grief counseling for sudden hearing loss and even progressive hearing loss. If you could tell me a little bit about your background and that and how you work with people.

Robin Chisholm-Seymour: Well, sure. Yes. My background is that I have a master's in counseling education from the University of Miami and my career began in Miami as a Substance Abuse Counselor. And that was the field I got into. I decided for a number of reasons not to get my doctorate. I kind of wanted to go another route. And I ended up moving to Atlanta and worked many, many years, both in the private and public sectors, in the mental health and psychiatric field. I have been doing actually a support group for 14 years at a local veterinary hospital for people who are grieving the loss of their pets. And that is another what I call under identified and under treated area. So that's something I do once a week.

Robin Chisholm-Seymour: As far as hearing loss goes over the years, I noticed in fact, many, many years ago, I started telling people that there's a psychological component to hearing loss. And you see that manifest in different ways. And again, as you asked me to everything I'm relating to is from either progressive as an adult or maybe older child, but progressive or sudden and hearing loss. And I realized that often people would say to me so and so blasts the TV and X, Y, Z. It's very frustrating. You have to yell at them. They don't understand what I'm saying, and they won't go get their hearing tested.

Robin Chisholm-Seymour: So that's one of the first cues that I had that something's going on. In other words, if you're losing your sight or you can't read something or can't see the television well, most of us, you have glasses, I have contacts and glasses. We go to the eye doctor. Usually, we don't put that off too long, but with hearing there's a resistance to getting tested. The second area is that over the years, I have done a lot of meeting and speaking with groups of people with hearing loss or groups of people in senior centers or senior living arrangements, senior neighborhoods. And I talk about hearing loss. One of my first questions always was, if you have hearing aids, are you wearing them? Are they in a drawer? And the show of hands was amazing how many had them but weren't wearing them. So that was another key.

Robin Chisholm-Seymour: Then the third thing for me that has become extremely apparent over the years, as I began to voluntarily support others with hearing loss as a volunteer, which I started formally doing in 2011, what I realized is in getting that cochlear implant the resistance of people in moving forward or even acknowledging they have an issue. The other piece of it is seeing so much anger and frustration from either people I talked to or online regarding either their hearing loss or how other people relate to them and don't support them. Or a lot of frustration if they get a cochlear implant, let's say anger and frustration focused on that process and a solution. All of these things, putting them together, I can't pinpoint the date that sort of the light bulb came on for me. But I started saying to people, we grieve the loss of our hearing. I hate to call them symptoms, but let's say behaviors that are being manifest are very much reflective of feeling and going through grief.

Richard: Is that the same as having an amputation? If somebody loses an arm or a leg, do they go through the grieving for the loss of that limb?

Robin Chisholm-Seymour: That's what I was going to say. Grief can be from loss of anything important to you. It can be loss of a loved one. It can be loss of a job. It can be loss of any of your senses or certainly body parts or functioning. If someone let's say becomes paralyzed, they've lost function. And of course, I add loss of pets and I know you've got your puppy there. A lot of people don't understand how deep that loss can be.

Richard: I've outlived four dogs so far. And the dog I have now is 15 and a half.

Robin Chisholm-Seymour: Oh.

Richard: I understand that part about the pets and the grieving.

Robin Chisholm-Seymour: As far as hearing loss goes, I've never done a formal study on this. I haven't kept notes through logs, but my observation over time, and a lot of what I do when I'm supporting people, is help them acknowledge and maybe even just identify that they're grieving that loss and that their feelings and behaviors are reflecting that.

Richard: A lot of the posts to my question, a number, not a lot, I think were in denial.

Robin Chisholm-Seymour: Yes.

Richard: They say I have family. I push my way through it. Now, men tend to do that a lot more than women. I understand that because men are not as bright as women. They hold a lot of stuff in. How do you deal with somebody who you feel is in denial?

Robin Chisholm-Seymour: There are several, they call them stages of grief and Elizabeth Kubler-Ross is the therapist that many years ago, penned these different stages of grief. They're not necessarily however stages that are sequential and you may not feel all of them, but denial is usually the first one and can be manifest in different ways. And the other two that I see the most to be honest is anger and depression. Okay? So those tend to go together. Someone may be feeling one and not everybody is depressed necessarily is anger or feels anger.

Robin Chisholm-Seymour: Yes, the start point generally in my observation, all these years is denial. And that feeds back to not getting help of any type. In other words, it may not even be going for an evaluation. It may be doing things every day to help yourself function better. A lot of that has to do with relating to other people and conversing and advocating yourself so that you can function better. If you're in denial, you're just sort of plowing through and not doing much about it. The denial piece is key. And the way to do that is really to kind of reach deep down and look at your feelings because oftentimes we have other people in our lives, family, and friends, to some degree that are pointing this out to us, but we don't want to hear it. Part of it is you have to open yourself up to that. And of course, it's painful.

Richard: You brought up a very important point because I've worked with couples through the Hearing Loss Association of America, the local chapter, and the unsupportive partner is the biggest problem that I've seen. They don't want to know anything about their partner's hearing loss. They don't want to cooperate in that. How often do you see that?

Robin Chisholm-Seymour: I can't say I've seen it be pervasive. I see some fabulous, significant others that are, and let me say this there's degrees of support. Okay? I will tell you my own case. My husband was extremely supportive through all of this with me, but one of the big things I hear people daily complain about, oh, my spouse still tries to talk to me from the other room or when they walk away or whatever, and they get angry about it. What I had to realize was, and we all do, hearing loss is invisible and yes, there are those of us who pay attention and remember, and always act accordingly. The majority of people don't, and it's not something personal. It's not that they're actively being non supportive. They just don't think about it. When I work with couples, try to get down to the degree of nonsupport.

Robin Chisholm-Seymour: And I actually was talking to a couple not long ago because when I do virtual sessions, let's say with candidates or recipients, I try to have the significant other there so that they're involved in it. But yes, I do run across cases where if you drill down to the degree of lack of support, some of it is other things going on in the relationship that is a whole other issue. Part of it is it's just easier not to deal with it. And part of it is the interaction between the two, because hearing loss affects both of you. It's part of working on that relationship, both in terms of how we, as those with hearing loss, relate to others and what our expectations are, but the other big, big piece of it is communicating and advocating for ourselves.

Robin Chisholm-Seymour:

And as an example, I'm 70, my mom is 89. She wears hearing aids. The biggest struggle I have with her, and I think it's generational, she is not good at communicating when she's not understanding something, and I can see it on her face. And I'll say, "Mom, did you get that?" And she won't do what I do, which is I'm sorry, I didn't understand that. Could you repeat it?

Richard: She bluffs.

Robin Chisholm-Seymour: Yeah. Getting back to the couples, if there is the feeling that one of the partners is non-supportive, a couple things have to happen. One is you have to drill down to what really is beneath all of that. And you have to look at the, like any relationship, and I'm not going to get off into marriage and relationship counseling, but communications has to be two-way. And often I find that the person with hearing loss is just making too many assumptions and expectations of that person rather than sitting down and saying, "This is really how we have to operate to do this." Does that make sense?

Richard: It makes perfect sense. I need to go back to one point though.
Robin Chisholm-Seymour: Okay.

Richard: Let's say you've had a sudden hearing loss and maybe you accept your grieving. What do you do at that point? How do you handle it? What steps do you take?

Robin Chisholm-Seymour: It depends on the individual to be honest. Acknowledging it is the first step. The next thing that I always suggest is action. Action always overrides a lot of times how you feel. Whatever that action plan might be for you, I mean, that's going to vary. In my case, I have to get up and do something. So that's when I started getting information. I joined the local, at the time that I since have started doing myself, but the local cochlear implant support group. I kept moving forward with action. And I didn't personally feel I needed counseling for it because even...

Richard: Denial.

Robin Chisholm-Seymour: I wasn't denying the issue. I knew I had lost my hearing, but my way of handling it works for me. Okay? Now that doesn't mean it works for everybody. Here's where counseling helps. That's where you need someone objective to listen, to understand, and often we use the term get it and then help you with dealing or coping with it.

Richard: That's a very important point. I want to discuss this. Okay. The type of counselor that you look for.

Robin Chisholm-Seymour: Right.

Richard: Some people would say life coach, other people would say, well, I want a counselor who has a hearing loss or understands hearing loss, which is very hard to find. The other one I found, I was very fortunate when I found a therapist who had survived leukemia, he had a death sentence and he survived that. He understood my loss. My question is how do you go about finding the help that you need?

Robin Chisholm-Seymour: And that's a challenging question. There's degrees. When you talk about a life coach, there are options. I mean, one is you can seek out support groups for this specific issue of yours, which we have now a good available choice among support groups. That's the kind of easiest one to feel you're with people who get it and understand. If you feel you need more intensive one on one attention for a while, and there are different types, I mean, a life coach is going to be someone that is encouraging and positive and helping you work out a game plan for yourself, an action plan. Counseling has different levels and definitions, and there are different even types of counselors or therapists.

Robin Chisholm-Seymour: There are licensed clinical social workers. There are people with my degree that are licensed clinical counselors. You can go up a notch to a licensed psychologist. That's going to make it more intense. But back to the question, most counselors will state that if they do grief counseling. Okay? I mean, they'll usually say the types of counseling because if they work with kids versus adults, or if they work with older adults and there's different styles of counseling, they usually advertise that. Now the challenge is sometimes finding the right one and we've had that challenge among the people in the pet loss group also.

Richard: You just triggered something. I wonder if calling the local funeral home would have a resource for grief counselors. I've never thought of doing that before.

Robin Chisholm-Seymour: I hadn't thought of that either, because usually nowadays with Google, what I usually suggest is that people start, if they have a primary care physician, usually that's the first person a lot of people talk to anyway, or their ENT or hearing clinic, whatever, whoever that is. Some of the ENT clinics will have some kind of relationship with a counselor or therapist, not all. But those are the ways that usually I suggest people start. It's hard to just pull out the yellow pages. Local support group, I would contact your local HLAA if there is other hearing related groups in your local area. And the other piece of it yes, is that when you contact someone, you really need to do initial due diligence and find out, like you did with the person who had had leukemia, get some background about them. Because grief counseling generally may focus more on either loss of human loved ones and, or losing your job, which can be prevalent over the years. That's not uncommon at all. Those are probably the two big ones.

Richard: Another question somebody posted or brought up to me was parents of pediatric cochlear implant recipients. The parent obviously goes into a panic at some point, but is that grief or is that loss of some sort, how would you interpret that?

Robin Chisholm-Seymour: Now I, first of all will say, I'm not a parent. So that may be someone to ask more of the parent. But being a parent is a whole different thing because that's going to be a myriad of feelings because your child is hurting and needs attention and care. So how much of it is grieving their loss of hearing versus the emotional stress of trying to help them is going to be different.

Robin Chisholm-Seymour: They're going to be kicking in that parent mode of what am I going to do to help whereas when I lost my hearing that morning, the only thing I thought about is I got to help myself. And I think that's where counseling can help if other levels of support, which also include, I mentioned the support groups, but if you have supportive family members and, of friends, or even through a support group, or even these online groups, now we have some mentors, of which I'm one. I don't formally counsel anybody, but a lot of it is providing support. And then if I feel they need, and I do this with pet loss too, if I feel they really need a more intensive level of care or attention, then I bring that in as a suggestion that they need to consider act on.

Richard: What about the progressive loss versus the sudden loss? You've seen the difference you've spoken to the differences. Do you want to address that a little bit?

Robin Chisholm-Seymour: Yes. And it is. And having lived through both of them, I can say how the different reactions were. The progressive to me can be more difficult in some ways, but also easier. And the progressive, you may be just building up your denial over time. And built into that though, what gets built into progressive is that unbeknownst to us, we are adapting. I honestly didn't wake up one day and say, "Oh, I'm going to start to read lips." I don't know when it started. I read lips pretty much proficiently, but I can't tell you, oh, when did you start? Or when did you go learn to read lips? The other things I learned to do over the years and because my hearing loss started, as yours, before we had as much technology as we do, had to learn to function as best we could.

Robin Chisholm-Seymour: Tied into progressive is our brain trying to make it work somehow. Now sometimes we get in our own way. With progressive over time, you've heard people say, "I'm doing just fine. I just turn the TV up. Or if I don't want to hear something, I just let it go. I don't care. I just nod." Right? Some of that in progressive, you know what you're doing, but you also are behaving in ways you may not be aware of. And so that can either tie into denial, or for me, it was always fuel to figure out a way to do what I wanted to do. I was working full time; I was having to travel for business and go through the airports and not hear what the pages said. I had no streaming. I had no mini mic. I had no nothing except texting on the phone, which wasn't big when I got started either. Right?

Robin Chisholm-Seymour: I had to with clients, tried to switch them to the written word, like emails and my, I hate to use the word excuse, but my explanation was to do business this information needs to be in writing. And I used that over the years. For progressive you either allow it to sink you more into denial or you use it to help figure out ways to get things done. With sudden, sudden puts you in a panic mode. You have to deal with that adrenaline rush and that sort of freaking out. And "Oh my gosh, what am I going to do?" Generally, there isn't denial as much when it's sudden until it kind of sinks in and you're having to deal with it and figure out what to do. And usually when it's sudden, that's when I see much more anger. I see much more the anger that kicks in and starts affecting all kinds of things. My family's not helping me. I can't understand when I go to the doctor, I can't work anymore, et cetera, et cetera.

Richard: Okay. You've covered a lot of ground and I'm sure your interview is going to be helpful to more people than you can imagine. But before we close off, I like to give you the opportunity to add to anything you would like to about the process of sudden hearing loss and how to handle it.

Robin Chisholm-Seymour: Well, first, I really appreciate this opportunity. When this came up, I was so excited because it is something that I've been sort of addressing quietly for a long time and it's near, and dear to me. What I would add definitely is take care of yourself and whatever you feel might work for you, even if it's baby steps, I'm a big proponent of action. And even if it's one small step, take a small step. Whether it's a phone call or an email or a text or Googling something to find out about it. Do something, because any small action gives you a sense of confidence and helps you move forward. Whereas I think we tend to feel overwhelmed with the big picture and that makes it harder to act, but just pick sort of one small thing and almost one every day. And that helps you move forward.

Richard: Robin, thank you so much for your time and your expertise. I really do appreciate it. And I'm sure that our listeners will too

Robin Chisholm-Seymour: Well, thank you so much, Richard, for the opportunity.

PART THREE

Rehabilitation Techniques

**NOTE: LIVE LINKS ARE FOUND AT
COCHLEARIMPLANTBASICS.COM**

Tips for Cochlear Implant and BAHA Rehabilitation

Your hearing journey begins the day of your activation. Though that first day of restored hearing is filled with much anticipation, emotion, and joy it is important to remember your hearing will most likely not be instantly "normal" nor equivalent to others' hearing experience. Just as no two people are alike, no two journeys into the world of cochlear implant hearing will be alike. What others have found helpful may not work for you. Some of these exercises require a helper (a hearing partner) to read and score your responses. <u>If you don't have a hearing partner on your journey, don't worry. Most of these suggestions can be done alone.</u>

NEVER COMPARE your hearing journey with that of others.

Many Cochlear Implant recipients will tell you that the **three P's – practice, patience, and perseverance-** will determine how well you hear. Please understand that having the mindset of "low expectations and high hopes" will spare you from disappointment and frustration during those early days of hearing.

Repetition, repetition, repetition!!!

Your hearing journey is ongoing your comprehension of speech and sounds will improve significantly over time. Learning to hear with a cochlear implant or BAHA is a skills development exercise like any other: the more you practice and commit to an exceptional hearing outcome, the better your hearing comprehension will improve. At times, this may be emotionally taxing and perhaps even frustrating, but recipients routinely create exceptional hearing outcomes by investing the required time and energy.

DO NOT GET DISCOURAGED. ATTITUDE IS 90% OF THE PATH TO SUCCESS.

This is a compilation of what other CI recipients, and I have found helpful in our hearing journeys.

- **Relax!!!** Your hearing journey is a marathon not a sprint. Just as an athlete conditions for her event you must also condition your brain to interpret the new sounds you're hearing.
- Do not set a timetable as to what and when you're going to understand the different sounds around you. Your listening comprehension will improve on a timeline that is unique to you.
- Let the sounds come to you.
- Look at everyday as a new day filled with **WOW** moments.
- Wear your processor all day. If you feel tired, overwhelmed by sound, or your hearing seems a little off it's fine to "rest "by taking off your processor for a short period of time. Giving your brain short breaks is just as beneficial as giving it a good workout.
- Close your eyes and take yourself to that "peaceful" place far away from the pressure to perfectly understand everything you hear.
- Keep the television or radio on all day. Using the wireless accessories will vastly improve sound. There will be no distortion nor interference from Wi-Fi networks, mobile phones, etc.
- Watch programs and movies with the subtitles but challenge yourself not to reply on the captioning exclusively. It's a good way to practice and will help with listening comprehension.
- YouTube has children's books with a reader. Storyonline.com is another excellent source for those beginning to rehab.

- Listen to audiobooks following along with the printed version of the book if helpful. Your local library may have an audiobook collection you can access for free.
- The Great Courses are lecture series on hundreds of topics. They may be found at your local library online. They are not closed captioned which forces you to lipread the lecturer while streaming the audio to your processor.
- Have someone read the newspaper or a passage from a book or poem and have you repeat it back to them.
- Have fun with your hearing rehab. Play games like name that sound. Enlist the help of family/friends to challenge you to name the sounds around you. Invent your own game.
- Listen to the radio (talk radio) when driving.
- If you don't have small children go to the park or playground to familiarize yourself with the way they speak.
- Have a child read to you or sing his/her favorite song. Children's voices can be just as difficult to understand as an adult's voice.
- Listen to music – easy listening/mellow – without a lot of instruments or vocals. Start by finding a song you remember following along with printed lyrics to jog your mental/listening memory. As you begin to understand music add different types of songs/music to your listening list. Hearmusicagain.com has helpful hints and easy listening internet music.
- Old songs may not sound like you remember them. In fact, they probably won't. Don't be discouraged. Your brain needs to learn to recognize them again. If the first time you listen to an old favorite, it sounds "off," play it again and again. Your brain will catch up to your ears! YouTube music

videos of familiar sounds will help. Search for your favorite song and add the words: with lyrics to your search term. You brain will kick in faster with the lyrics and the music together. Remember, even people with normal hearing often have problems with understanding the lyrics. Patience will pay off.

- Music with more rhythm tends to be easier to learn. In the beginning, jazz with a lot of brass, is the easiest way to get music to sound recognizable and normal.

- Set up times to call family members and friends to hold a phone conversation every day.

- Go for a walk or sit outside to re-acclimate or learn the sounds of nature. Try to pick out the different songs that birds sing. Soon those songs will be in perfect harmony.

- Go to restaurants at non-peak times.

- Turn on appliances such as the microwave, dishwasher, washer, dryer etc. Put your ear close to anything around the house just to learn the sound.

- Utilize your wireless accessories. They can be a big help in various situations (car, restaurant, etc.) Each manufacturer offers their own set of devices. Do your research. When doing rehabilitation exercises from a laptop or television, direct streaming of the sound source is preferred.

- Sit at the front of the room to hear/see the speaker. Don't be shy. If you cannot hear a speaker at a lecture or in a classroom, ask them to clip a remote mic accessory to their shirt or jacket. It will make the experience much more enjoyable. Just don't forget to get it back at the end.

- Use a T-Coil setting to help you hear in venues that are equipped with the hearing loop.

- Use your remote assistant. Adjust the volume and sensitivity for different hearing environments. Your audiologist can help you select settings that are suitable for your lifestyle and interests. Remember again, no two people have the same loss or the same solution for their hearing journey. Everyone can have a customized solution.

- **Think outside the box!!!** There is so much you can do to connect the dots to hearing. Just use your imagination.

- **Other helpful ideas:**

- Keep a journal of both good and bothersome issues you encounter. Take that journal to your appointments with your audiologist. This specific feedback will provide your audiologist a better understanding of the problems you may be experiencing positively influence adjustments.

- Work with your audiologist to improve the fine tuning. Ask about T (threshold levels – softest sounds you hear) and C levels (comfort levels – loudest sounds you can comfortably tolerate). Discuss the different programs/coding strategies and when to use them. Learn as much as you can about the process and the features available to your processor.

- Manufacturers recommend that you change your microphone covers once every three months or sooner if you live in an area where humidity is high, you perspire often or notice a change in sound quality. Keeping clean microphone covers in place is important.

- Ideally, store your processor in a dryer such as a Zephyr or other drying device, every night. If your device has a replaceable desiccant cartridge be sure to mark the date on it and replace as per the instructions. REMEMBER: Moisture is the enemy of all electronics.

- If you use them, recharge your rechargeable batteries, and keep those not in use in the recharger unit.

USEFUL REHABILITATION PROGRAMS AND SUPPORT

NOTE: LIVE LINKS ARE FOUND AT COCHLEARIMPLANTBASICS.COM

- TED Talks www.ted.com/talks
- News in Easy English newsineasyenglish.com News in Easy English – Easy News for ESL Listening newsineasyenglish.com
- App called **Speech Banana**
- Practice phone calls with a family member or friend
- Audiobooks along with a print copy
- App called **Hear Coach**
- App called Nature Sounds
- App called **Breethe**
- App called **Coffitivity**
- App called **Mondly** for different languages
- App called **TOEIC** for English as a second language
- **Angel Sounds Interactive Listening Rehabilitation & Hearing test**:
- http://angelsound.tigerspeech.com/

Aural Rehabilitation Resource Guide is another excellent source of programs, some free and others for sale. Aural-rehabiliation.pdf(unc.edu)

Facebook groups offer support for recipients of all ages. Some groups to consider are:

- Cochlear Implant Daily Rehab
- Bilateral CI Warrior
- Cochlear Awareness Network
- Cochlear Implant Users
- Cochlear Hybrid Implant Group
- Cochlear Implant Experiences
- Cochlear Implants How to Enjoy Music
- Podcast interviews at cochlearimplantbasics.com

These programs are produced by different cochlear implant manufacturers but may be utilized by other cochlear implant brand recipients.

COCHLEAR

- Communications Center
- http://www.cochlear.com/wps/wcm/connect/us/communica tion-corner

For a comprehensive Cochlear rehabilitation program, ask your Cochlear representative for the Adult-Home Based Hearing Therapy Manual (publication FUN3570 ISS2 Dept 20)

MED-EL

Rehab at home for adults' series

https://blog.medel.com/category/tips-tricks/rehab-at-home-posts/

Med-El Mondays aural rehabilitation small group zoom meetings.

They rotate topics each month, so all the topics show up and aural rehab is one of the topics.)

https://web.cvent.com/event/15c20e19-df0c-4dd7-b47f-2193f55b450b/regProcessStep1

Med-El adult rehabilitation kits to use with a family member or friend.

https://blog.medel.pro/introducing-medel-adult-rehabilitation-kits/

One on one captioned zoom meetings with a Med-El audiologist to help guide aural rehabilitation (aural rehab is one of the topics to select when registering for the free time slot)

https://web.cvent.com/event/9f87401e-5bd8-4868-9e78-1fbba262e086/regProcessStep1

https://www.medel.com/support/rehab/rehabilitation-downloads

https://www.medel.com/support/rehab

Music For Cochlear Implant Users: MED-EL's Spotify Playlists - The MED-EL Blog (medel.com)

ADVANCED BIONICS

- https://hearingsuccess.com
- https://play.google.com/store/apps/details?id=com.advanced bionics.wordsuccess&hl=en_US&gl=US
- https://thelisteningroom.com
- https://www.advancedbionics.com/us/en/home/ab4kids/tool s-for-schools.html

Some Closing Comments about Rehabilitation

One of the most common areas of concern that candidates for a cochlear implant mention is rehabilitation. How much time is required for sounds to normalize? How many hours a day will they need to do it? What if they live alone and do not have a "hearing partner" to assist them. What programs are available?

All hearing journeys are unique. That also applies to rehabilitation. In rare cases, at activation, it all sounds normal. These "rockstar" activations are heartwarming, but most of us require effort to hear sounds as we remember.

Robin Chisholm Seymour's observation about rehabilitation says it best:

"Although I do recognize and appreciate the existence of specialized apps and tools that are now available to recipients, I strongly believe that real life listening is necessary. My suggestion is that it is so important to think about what you wanted to get cochlear implants and how being able to hear can impact your life in terms of work, interests, communications, etc. Not only are our CI learning journeys unique, but our motivations and goals are as well, as our interests and needs.

That being said, I've shared before that I got my first CI in early 2010, and there was no social media like today. We did not have wireless streaming with or without an accessory or hardware and we did not have any apps.

My personal goal was and continues to be that I live my life as normally and as fully as I used to prior to my hearing loss. I am not willing to compromise or give up anything in my life as a result of hearing challenges. My definition of those words, "rehabilitation" or "practice", is much broader than in sometimes used. I believe that our brain has to learn to hear with the CI and has to learn to hear it within those environments that we are going to experience within the contents of our needs and interest.

What I did and continue to do is wear my Cis during all waking hours and in all hearing environments that I want to experience. The only streaming I do at all is to use the phone, which I do extremely easily and pretty much all day long. I don't use headphones. I don't use an accessory, and I do occasionally stream music. But I went from not being able to listen to music at all prior to my Cis, to pushing through music. Music sounded terrible. Gradually, overtime, it improved to the point that I now listen to music directly through whatever source is, radio, CD's and concerts, etc.

I had to hit the ground running after my first CI and that included working, volunteering, and most important horse shows which were extremely noisy as you can imagine. Going to dinner in a noisy restaurant at a huge table with 25 people obviously was challenging, but I still did it.

My learning to hear with my CI's. Has been challenging. Daily listening and exposing myself to the world sounds and speech, no matter initially how challenging it was. Because after my first CI I had no speech or sound or understanding at all. My audiologist gave me pages and pages of exercises to do, but those were list of individual words to practice with another person with a mouth covered so I could learn individual words. We graduated to simple sentences.

I know that this can be done with an app, but I was listening to real voices rather than streaming. Having tools now. To help. With learning to hear with the CIs are wonderful. But it's also important to keep in mind it's going to take more than a couple of hours a day of rehab or practice with an app to get to feeling functional and comfortable out in the everyday world. My suggestions are to always identify your hearing goals, your life goals, and then adapt any learning strategy to those goals. They worked for me.

Kelly Flodin, another cochlear implant recipient, reiterated Robin's observations:

"I agree with Robin that real life, real world listening, in all the environments we find ourselves in, is the best rehab for CIs. I consider anything we listen to as rehab. We want to hear what goes on around us in real life every day so actual practicing is critical, in my opinion.

I've had my CIs for a little over two years. Early on I would just listen to the world around me and try tracking down and identifying anything I could hear. I got speech recognition pretty quickly. Conversations were the best for that."

Made in the USA
Las Vegas, NV
01 December 2023

81938671R00223